Thyroid Cancer and Nuclear Accidents

Thyroid Cancer and Nuclear Accidents

Long-Term Aftereffects of Chernobyl and Fukushima

Edited by

Shunichi Yamashita
Nagasaki University, Nagasaki, Japan
Fukushima Medical University, Fukushima, Japan

Gerry Thomas
Imperial College, London, United Kingdom

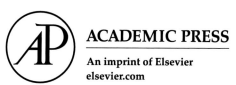

ACADEMIC PRESS

An imprint of Elsevier
elsevier.com

Academic Press is an imprint of Elsevier
125 London Wall, London EC2Y 5AS, United Kingdom
525 B Street, Suite 1800, San Diego, CA 92101-4495, United States
50 Hampshire Street, 5th Floor, Cambridge, MA 02139, United States
The Boulevard, Langford Lane, Kidlington, Oxford OX5 1GB, United Kingdom

British Library Cataloguing-in-Publication Data
A catalogue record for this book is available from the British Library

Library of Congress Cataloging-in-Publication Data
A catalog record for this book is available from the Library of Congress

ISBN: 978-0-12-812768-1

For Information on all Academic Press publications
visit our website at https://www.elsevier.com/books-and-journals

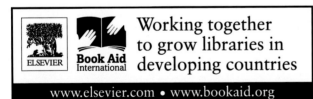

Working together
to grow libraries in
developing countries

ELSEVIER   Book Aid
            International

www.elsevier.com • www.bookaid.org

Publisher: Mica Haley
Acquisition Editor: Rafael E. Teixeira
Editorial Project Manager: Timothy Bennett
Production Project Manager: Priya Kumaraguruparan
Cover Designer: Matthew Limbert

Typeset by MPS Limited, Chennai, India

CONTENTS

LIST OF CONTRIBUTORS

Masafumi Abe
Fukushima Medical University, Fukushima, Japan

Hyeong-Sik Ahn
Korea University, Seoul, Korea

Johannes Biko
University of Würzburg, Würzburg, Germany

Tetiana Bogdanova
V.P. Komisarenko Institute of Endocrinology and Metabolism of National Academy of Medical Sciences of Ukraine, Kyiv, Ukraine

John D. Boice Jr.
National Council on Radiation Protection and Measurements, Bethesda, MD, United States; Vanderbilt University School of Medicine, Nashville, TN, United States

Andre Bouville
National Cancer Institute, Rockville, MD, United States

Igor Branovan
Project Chernobyl, Brooklyn, NY, United States

Alina Brenner
National Cancer Institute, Rockville, MD, United States

Svitlana Burko
V.P. Komisarenko Institute of Endocrinology and Metabolism of National Academy of Medical Sciences of Ukraine, Kyiv, Ukraine

Stephen Chanock
National Cancer Institute, Rockville, MD, United States

Sergey Chekin
A. Tsyb MRRC, Obninsk, Russia

Malcolm Crick
Secretariat of the United Nations Scientific Committee on the Effects of Atomic Radiation (UNSCEAR), Vienna, Austria

Ivan I. Dedov
Endocrine Research Centre, Moscow, Russian Federation

Tetiana Dekhtyarova
V.P. Komisarenko Institute of Endocrinology and Metabolism of
National Academy of Medical Sciences of Ukraine, Kyiv, Ukraine

Yuri E. Demidchik
Republican Centre for Thyroid Tumors, Minsk, Belarus; Belarusian
Medical Academy of Postgraduate Education, Minsk, Belarus

Valentina M. Drozd
The International Fund "Help for Patients with Radiation-Induced
Thyroid Cancer "Arnica", Minsk, Belarus; Belarusian Medical
Academy of Postgraduate Education, Minsk, Belarus

Vladimir Drozdovitch
National Cancer Institute, Rockville, MD, United States

Mikhail V. Fridman
Minsk Municipal Clinical Oncological Dispensary, Minsk, Belarus;
Republican Centre for Thyroid Tumors, Minsk, Belarus

Vsevolod Galkin
A. Tsyb MRRC, Obninsk, Russia

Abel J. González
Argentine Nuclear Regulatory Authority, Buenos Aires, Argentina

Tamara Gulii
V.P. Komisarenko Institute of Endocrinology and Metabolism of
National Academy of Medical Sciences of Ukraine, Kyiv, Ukraine

Maureen Hatch
National Cancer Institute, Rockville, MD, United States

Tetsuo Ishikawa
Fukushima Medical University, Fukushima, Japan;
Hiroshima University, Hiroshima, Japan

Viktor Ivanov
A. Tsyb MRRC, Obninsk, Russia

Kenji Kamiya
Fukushima Medical University, Fukushima, Japan; Hiroshima
University, Hiroshima, Japan

Andrey Kaprin
NMRRC, Obninsk, Russia

Valerii Kashcheev
A. Tsyb MRRC, Obninsk, Russia

Polina Kashcheeva
A. Tsyb MRRC, Obninsk, Russia

Hyun-Jung Kim
Korea University, Seoul, Korea

Elena Kochergina
A. Tsyb MRRC, Obninsk, Russia

Aleksandr Korelo
A. Tsyb MRRC, Obninsk, Russia

Olga Krasko
National Academy of Sciences of Belarus, Minsk, Belarus

Alfred K. Lam
Griffith University, Gold Coast, QLD, Australia

Ilya Likhtarev
National Scientific Center of Radiation Medicine, Kyiv, Ukraine

Mark P. Little
National Cancer Institute, Rockville, MD, United States

Kiyohiko Mabuchi
National Cancer Institute, Rockville, MD, United States

Marat Maksioutov
A. Tsyb MRRC, Obninsk, Russia

Svetlana Mankovskaya
Republican Centre for Thyroid Tumors, Minsk, Belarus; National Academy of Sciences of Belarus, Minsk, Belarus

Takashi Matsuzuka
Fukushima Medical University, Fukushima, Japan

Alexandr Menyajlo
A. Tsyb MRRC, Obninsk, Russia

Sanae Midorikawa
Fukushima Medical University, Fukushima, Japan

Jaya Mohan
Secretariat of the United Nations Scientific Committee on the Effects
of Atomic Radiation (UNSCEAR), Vienna, Austria

Pavel Moiseev
Republican Scientific Practical Centre of Oncology and Medical
Radiology named after N.N. Aleksandrov, Minsk, Belarus

Shigenobu Nagataki
Nagasaki University, Nagasaki, Japan

Hitoshi Ohto
Fukushima Medical University, Fukushima, Japan

Akira Ohtsuru
Fukushima Medical University, Fukushima, Japan

Valeriy Oliynyk
V.P. Komisarenko Institute of Endocrinology and Metabolism of
National Academy of Medical Sciences of Ukraine, Kyiv, Ukraine

Tamara Platonova
The International Fund "Help for Patients with Radiation-Induced
Thyroid Cancer "Arnica", Minsk, Belarus

Christoph Reiners
University of Würzburg, Würzburg, Germany

Tatiana I. Rogounovitch
Nagasaki University, Nagasaki, Japan

Pavel O. Rumiantsev
Endocrine Research Centre, Moscow, Russian Federation

Vladimir A. Saenko
Nagasaki University, Nagasaki, Japan

Kurt W. Schmid
University of Duisburg-Essen, Essen, Germany

Natalia Seleva
A. Tsyb MRRC, Obninsk, Russia

Natalia Shchukina
A. Tsyb MRRC, Obninsk, Russia

Nikolay Shiglik
Project Chernobyl, Brooklyn, NY, United States

Hiroki Shimura
Fukushima Medical University, Fukushima, Japan

Victor Shpak
V.P. Komisarenko Institute of Endocrinology and Metabolism of
National Academy of Medical Sciences of Ukraine, Kyiv, Ukraine

Iwao Sugitani
Nippon Medical School, Tokyo, Japan

Satoru Suzuki
Fukushima Medical University, Fukushima, Japan

Shinichi Suzuki
Fukushima Medical University School of Medicine, Fukushima, Japan

Koichi Tanigawa
Fukushima Medical University, Fukushima, Japan

Valeriy Tereshchenko
V.P. Komisarenko Institute of Endocrinology and Metabolism of
National Academy of Medical Sciences of Ukraine, Kyiv, Ukraine

Gerry Thomas
Imperial College London, London, United Kingdom

Mykola Tronko
V.P. Komisarenko Institute of Endocrinology and Metabolism of
National Academy of Medical Sciences of Ukraine, Kyiv, Ukraine

Konstantin Tumanov
A. Tsyb MRRC, Obninsk, Russia

Oleg Vlasov
A. Tsyb MRRC, Obninsk, Russia

Laryssa Voskoboynyk
V.P. Komisarenko Institute of Endocrinology and Metabolism of
National Academy of Medical Sciences of Ukraine, Kyiv, Ukraine

Wolfgang Weiss
Federal Office for Radiation Protection, Emmendingen, Germany

Shunichi Yamashita
Nagasaki University, Nagasaki, Japan

Galyna Zamotayeva
V.P. Komisarenko Institute of Endocrinology and Metabolism of
National Academy of Medical Sciences of Ukraine, Kyiv, Ukraine

Liudmyla Zurnadzhy
V.P. Komisarenko Institute of Endocrinology and Metabolism of
National Academy of Medical Sciences of Ukraine, Kyiv, Ukraine

Thirty Years After Chernobyl and 5 After Fukushima—What Have We Learnt and What Do We Still Need to Know?

Gerry Thomas[1] and Shunichi Yamashita[2]
[1]Imperial College London, London, United Kingdom [2]Nagasaki University, Nagasaki, Japan

INTRODUCTION

The year 2016 saw the anniversaries of two accidents at nuclear power plants that resulted in exposure to radiation in fallout of populations living in their immediate vicinity—the 30th anniversary of the Chernobyl accident in 1986 and the fifth anniversary of the Fukushima accident in 2011. A meeting was held in Fukushima city in September 2016 to ask the question: "What do we know and what do we need to learn from these two accidents?"(Saenko et al., 2017). This book serves as a record of the presentations made by experts from the medical community, both inside and outside Japan, and from those international bodies charged with providing guidance for response in these types of emergencies to protect local populations from the harmful effects of radiation. One of the key lessons that we still need to learn, as evidenced from the expert reports on both accidents by the WHO, UNSCEAR, and IAEA (UNSCEAR Report to the General Assembly of the United Nations, 2008; WHO report on health risk assessment from the nuclear accident after the, 2011; UNSCEAR report, 2013; IAEA report, 2015) is how to get the balance right between protection of the public from actual health effects caused by the direct interaction with radiation on the tissues of the body, and protection of the public from the fear of radiation.

THE RELATIONSHIP BETWEEN DOSE AND RESPONSE

There is a common misconception that exposure to radiation from a nuclear power plant accident is (1) different from exposure to natural background radiation or medical radiation and (2) that the dose to an individual is much greater than it is. Health effects from any hazardous substance, termed a toxin (and radiation is essentially a toxic agent), are related to the dose to which an individual is exposed. We understand dose when we talk about chemical agents and it is widely accepted that in small doses some chemicals, e.g., therapeutic agents such as acetaminophen (paracetamol), are beneficial to our health. We also accept that taken in excess (i.e., at high doses) the health effects can be detrimental. In the case of paracetamol, doses of between 1−4 g/day may be safely ingested for protracted periods of time with no deleterious effect on human health. However, a single dose of 7.5−10 g, which is only twice that of the recommended maximum daily dose, is likely to result in significant liver toxicity within 24−48 h and potentially death, unless appropriate medical care is swiftly administered. Paracetamol represents a toxin that we are content to trust at small individual doses, even when we voluntarily expose ourselves to it over a protracted time period, yet we know it has potential fatal consequences when exposure is to a high single exposure. In the United Kingdom it is the most common agent of intentional self-harm. Between 2000−08 there were 90−155 deaths from paracetamol poisoning every year (Hawton et al., 2011). In addition, there are deaths resulting from paracetamol compounds. It is the most common cause of acute liver failure.

However, we seem to lose the understanding of the relationship between dose and effect that we have with other toxins when it comes to radiation. Perhaps this is because calculating the dose for radiation exposure is complicated.

There are different types of radiation, but the one type that concerns us here is ionizing. Ionizing radiation is radiation that carries enough energy that it can ionize atoms or molecules (i.e., strip electrons from them) as it passes through matter. It can come in two forms—waves, which are uncharged, or particles, that carry either a positive or negative charge. Radioactive elements produce several different types of radiation and this can also be of different levels of energy. Wave forms of radiation can penetrate through a body, and not all of the waves will necessarily interact with the tissue in your body as the wave passes through—believe it or not a lot of your body is space! Particulate forms of radiation penetrate less because they are charged, and usually need to be ingested or inhaled to deliver a dose of radiation to the body's cells. All radioactive isotopes have a given physical half-life—the time it takes to release half of the radioactivity present. All radioactive isotopes are also chemical elements, and chemicals have a biological half life (the time taken for half of a given amount of the chemical to be excreted from the body) that it is dependent on their solubility and whether they are taken up and bound by particular tissues. The dose received internally by the body from a given amount of a radioactive isotope is a function of both biological and physical half life—in most cases where physical half-life is much longer than biological half-life, the dose to individual tissues within the body is small. The internal dose is probably the most important one to consider when we are trying to understand the health effects of low doses of radiation.

In medicine we use X-rays for diagnosis; the exposure to the atomic bombs was primarily gamma radiation—both of these are wave forms of radiation. The exposure from nuclear power plant accidents is predominantly particulate (alpha and beta), but some radioactive elements also release gamma radiation, so the dose to which a person is exposed becomes a combination of different types of radiation, making calculation of the dose and advice for radiation protection more difficult.

We are all exposed to radiation in small doses over a protracted period of time. Individually, our average annual dose to background radiation is around 2 mSv, but this does vary worldwide considerably up to 10 mSv/year, with some individuals in Ramsar, Iran, receiving 260 mSv/year. It is estimated that the average Japanese would be exposed to 170 mSv of radiation from background alone during their lifetime. Individuals living in the highest areas of background radiation show no discernible effects on their health (Hendry et al., 2009).

DOSE AND HEALTH RISKS ASSOCIATED WITH RADIATION EXPOSURE

We know from studies of survivors of the Atomic bombs in Japan that high doses of radiation are associated with an increased risk of cancer. However, the problem comes when we try to attribute risk to doses of radiation below 100 mSv (it should be noted that this is 100 mSv in addition to a lifetime exposure to background radiation levels). Our health is affected by a great many other factors in addition to radiation exposure. To put this into context, if Americans were given a single dose of 100 mSv of radiation each, one individual in 100 would be expected to develop cancer (solid cancer or leukemia) from radiation, while approximately 42 of the 100 individuals would be expected to develop solid cancer or leukemia from other causes. Lower doses would produce proportionally lower risks. For example, it is theoretically predicted that approximately one individual in 1000 would develop cancer from an exposure to 10 mSv, whereas 420 would develop cancer from other causes (Committee to Assess Health Risks from Exposure to Low Levels of Ionizing Radiation, 2006). From these figures obtained from many assumptions you can see clearly how difficult it becomes to attribute radiation as a cause of cancer in a given exposed population as the dose decreases.

It is known that children are more sensitive to toxins, including radiation. This is related to their small body and organ size, but also in the case of carcinogens to the fact that their organs are still growing. It is widely accepted that exposure to agents that can damage and alter DNA structure (such as radiation) are more effective when cells in a tissue are undergoing cell division. Biologically the balance between DNA damage and repair maintains its genetic homeostasis and determines cell fate. At high doses agents that can alter DNA structure make very useful therapeutic agents for cancer—ironically at low doses the same agents do not cause enough DNA alterations in normal tissue to result in cell death, but sufficient to enable mutated cells to survive and divide, potentially resulting in cancer in the long term.

WHAT HAVE WE LEARNT FROM CHERNOBYL?

So what have we learnt from Chernobyl and can this inform us about what we should expect in terms of health effects from the Fukushima accident? Firstly, it should be noted that these two accidents where quite different in character. One happened at a time in history when it was still possible to hide what was happening in a rural area of a secretive country, the other happened in full view of the world's press in an urbanized area, at a time when it takes seconds for information to travel around the globe. The two accidents were different in terms of magnitude, with Fukushima releasing 10% of the radiation released at Chernobyl. Radiation doses to the workers on site at the time of the accident and in the immediate aftermath were significantly different. A total of 134 first responders were exposed to doses of over 1 Sv (1000 mSv) and developed acute radiation syndrome

(ARS) at Chernobyl, and 28 subsequently died as a direct consequence of their exposure within a matter of months of the accident.
At Fukushima, only six workers received doses of radiation above
250 mSv; the highest dose was 650 mSv, substantially lower than the
threshold for ARS (IAEA report, 2015). This book focuses only on
what we can learn from Chernobyl about the likely effects on the
health of the general population, rather than on what we can learn
about any potential health effects to those working at the power
plants themselves. It is divided into sections with the first four chapters covering the history of the Chernobyl accident from the perspective of the regulatory bodies involved in radiation protection. The
second section (Chapters 5–12) focuses on the single radiobiological
consequence of the Chernobyl accident, thyroid cancer in those who
were young at exposure. The third section (Chapters 13–20) focuses
on the Fukushima accident.

Volatile radioactive isotopes of iodine and cesium were released at
both accidents. We had learnt after Chernobyl that inhalation and
ingestion of these isotopes were of concern to the general population
living in the vicinity of the nuclear power plants. To avoid inhalation, the population in the vicinity of Fukushima Dai-ichi was
advised to evacuate and shelter indoors. Internal thyroid doses to
Fukushima residents are retrospectively under evaluation and mostly
estimated to be lower than 30 mSv (Kim et al., 2016). To avoid
ingestion, the Japanese government acted swiftly to cut the food
chain and thus remove exposure from radioiodine via the consumption of contaminated green leafy vegetables and milk. All the contaminated foods were immediately disposed of. These actions, plus
the fact that the radiation released was 90% lower, resulted in very
low radiation doses to the population (see Chapter 13: A Review of
Studies on Thyroid Dose Estimation After the Fukushima Accident)
compared with Chernobyl, both at the whole body and critically at
the thyroid level. The estimated lifetime dose from the Fukushima
accident to 95% of the residents in that area is estimated to be 5 mSv
(see Chapter 20: The Radiological Consequences of the Fukushima
Dai'ichi NPP Accident: Estimates From the Group of Experts
Convened by the International Atomic Energy Agency).

The accident at Chernobyl happened just prior to a political
sea-change in the USSR, and Chapter 2, Thirty Years After
the Chernobyl Nuclear Power Plant Accident: Contribution From

Japan—"Confirming the Increase of Childhood Thyroid Cancer," serves as a firsthand history of how this affected the response of those based outside the USSR to the accident. As stated in Chapter 1, Thirty Years After Chernobyl—Overview of the Risks of Thyroid Cancer, Based Upon the UNSCEAR Scientific Reports (2008—12), the only health effect directly attributable to exposure to radioactive isotopes in fallout from the accident is, and remains to this day, thyroid cancer in those who were children at the time of exposure. It was clear 4—5 years after the Chernobyl accident that exposure to radioiodine had resulted in an increase in thyroid cancer in children in the regions of present-day Belarus, Ukraine, and Russia that were closest to the accident site. This is reviewed in Chapters 5—9.

It is still a common opinion amongst the lay public that a cancer diagnosis ultimately means a cancer death. This could not be further from the truth, particularly with respect to thyroid cancer. Our ability to detect ever-smaller lesions using highly sensitive medical equipment has led to the detection of some cancers that would never have become clinically apparent and are no threat to life. Some organs of the body, such as the thyroid, appear to have the ability to produce minute lesions that become stalled in their ability to develop the characteristics of a life-threatening malignancy, namely local invasion and the ability to spread to other parts of the body, seed and grow. It is estimated that the old methods of manual palpation of the thyroid resulted in a detection rate of 2%—6%. Ultrasonography of the neck raises the detection rate to 19%—35%, and careful sectioning of the thyroid post-mortem raises the frequency still further to 8%—65% (Dean and Gharib, 2008). Any oncologist will inform you that if a lesion remains within its tissue of origin and does not exhibit expansile growth such that it exerts pressure on key structures within that tissue, or secrete factors that destabilize the body's homeostasis, it is very unlikely to result in your death. Experience with using sensitive screening methods to detect small thyroid cancers in other situations has shown that finding thyroid cancer earlier does not result in better outcomes and reduce mortality (see Chapter 17: Thyroid Cancer Screening and Overdiagnosis in Korea). Therefore, the benefit and risk of early diagnosis of thyroid cancer in children should be carefully reevaluated, as a result of the experience of the thyroid screening program post Fukushima, especially in regard to the implementation and continuation of mass screening using highly sophisticated ultrasound equipment. Screening also causes problems in attributing a rising incidence of a disease to a specific cause, leading to an overestimation of the actual increase (see Chapter 4: Reassessing the Capability to Attribute Pediatric Thyroid Cancer to Radiation Exposure: The FHMS Experience and Chapter 15: The Features of Childhood and Adolescent Thyroid Cancer After the Fukushima Nuclear Power Plant Accident).

It is critical to balance the risks of treatment against the risks that the cancer poses if left untreated, or overdiagnosis is converted to over-treatment. Thyroid cancer is relatively easy to treat using surgery (see Chapter 15: The Features of Childhood and Adolescent Thyroid Cancer After the Fukushima Nuclear Power Plant Accident) followed by high doses of radioiodine to kill any remaining cells not removed by the surgery (see Chapter 11: Results of Treatment in Children and Adolescents With Differentiated Thyroid Carcinoma Not Exposed and Exposed to Radiation From the Chernobyl Accident and Chapter 18: Management of Papillary Thyroid Carcinoma in Japan). It is ironic that we have the best targeted treatment of any cancer type in radioiodine for thyroid cancer because of the unique ability of the thyroid cell to concentrate iodine. At high doses this results in the death of the cell, but at much lower doses, particularly in children, exposure to the same agent can result in an increased risk of thyroid cancer. As with any cancer, a better understanding of the biology that drives the cancer has the potential to lead to better tailored treatment and outcomes for the patient. The ability to be able to study the thyroid cancers that have arisen following the Chernobyl accident has led to a far better understanding of thyroid cancer in general, and has shown that thyroid cancer in the child may be driven by different molecular biology than the same cancer in older patients. This is not something that is unique to thyroid cancer, and is an area of research that shows huge promise in being able to give better information on prognosis, but also to advise on personalizing treatment to the individual cancer and patient (see Chapter 12: Somatic Genomics of Childhood Thyroid Cancer). Ultimately it may mean that by combining clinical and molecular features of cancer, less invasive surgery or less toxic adjuvant treatment can be offered to the patient based on sound scientific evidence, thus improving a patient's quality of life post their cancer diagnosis.

WHAT SHOULD WE LEARN FROM FUKUSHIMA?

The Chernobyl accident has provided us with a plethora of scientific data that needs to be reviewed in order to refine our response to future accidents at nuclear power plant accidents. Some of the lessons were learnt well—the need to reduce inhalation of contaminated air and ingestion of contaminated food, and understanding that the only health consequence from exposure to the radiation was likely to be thyroid cancer by an initial internal exposure of radioiodines in the young. Perhaps the most important lesson we still need to learn comes from our reaction and mentality to the Fukushima accident. This accident was the first to happen in the full glare of the media spotlight, and in the age of social media. There must have been huge pressure to be seen to act, and the accident was compounded by the physical effects on the affected communities of a massive earthquake followed by a tsunami that resulted in around 20,000 deaths. It is easy therefore to understand why the immediate response was evacuation. However, prolonged exclusion from well-established communities has led to huge emotional and psychological issues (Ando, 2016). Moving the frail and ill without proper planning and support led to more than 1000 deaths (Hasegawa et al., 2016). These deaths are not attributable to the radiation itself but more to the process and the results of evacuation as a result of the fear of the radiation. That fear was not helped by the reaction of the press, fueled by scaremongering by pseudoscientists, to the reports of the Fukushima accident. In order to seek to allay fears, the government established a wide-reaching health management survey in Fukushima (Yasumura et al., 2012). However, surveys are not primarily scientific studies (see Chapter 3: From Chernobyl to Fukushima and Beyond—A Focus on Thyroid Cancer). Health and wellbeing is affected by a very large number of factors and to attribute any health effect to a particular cause careful scientific studies that involve control groups to take account of confounding factors are required. These usually take the form of epidemiological studies (see Chapter 8: Thyroid Cancer Risk in Ukraine Following the Chernobyl Accident (The Ukrainian—American Cohort Thyroid Study)). These require time and identification that something has changed in the population exposed to a given environmental agent. To link exposure to that environmental agent requires careful selection of cases and controls to be able to identify causality. Explaining the difference between surveys and studies to the general public is not easy, particularly where this involves using sensitive screening methods. Chapter 16, Psychosocial Impact of the Thyroid Examination of the Fukushima Health Management Survey, focuses on the psychosocial effects of mounting a screening study and the problems of misinterpretation of the data it generates.

So what have we learnt from these two accidents? Firstly that exposure to radioactive iodine in fallout can cause thyroid cancer in those who are youngest at exposure. In contrast, exposure to radioactive cesium appears to have no discernible effect on the health of the general population. The magnitude of the health effects is related to the dose of radiation and simple measures can reduce the dose to the individual, and therefore the risk to health. We can set up surveys with the best of intentions, but it is extremely difficult to communicate what the results really mean to the survey subjects, their immediate family, the general population, and the world's press. The fact that the Fukushima accident is likely to result in no discernible health effects from radiation (see Chapter 19: UNSCEAR Activities Related to the 2011 Fukushima-Daiichi Nuclear Power Station Accident), yet our immediate actions to evacuate the area, and prevent people returning to areas of land that have levels of radiation post the accident that are lower than many areas of the globe have naturally, have led to deaths and huge psychological effects to the detriment of quality of life. These facts should make us question whether we need to rethink our policies on radiation protection. We seem to have become so focused on a single risk to health that, in the grand scheme of things, pales into insignificance when we look at the effects of lifestyle factors such as smoking and obesity on our health. Should this not give us pause for thought? Surely it is our duty as scientists to learn from our mistakes and provide an evidence base that policy makers can use to protect future generations?

Finally, three of the contributors to this volume have sadly passed away in the few months since our meeting was held. Professor Shigenobu Nagataki, the author of Chapter 2, Thirty Years After the Chernobyl Nuclear Power Plant Accident: Contribution From Japan—"Confirming the Increase of Childhood Thyroid Cancer," made a huge contribution to thyroid research in general, and the study of post-Chernobyl thyroid cancer in particular. Prof. Yuri Demidchik has just passed away. He was an excellent thyroid surgeon and the first author of Chapter 5, Post-Chernobyl Pediatric Papillary Thyroid Carcinoma in Belarus: Histopathological Features, Treatment Strategy, and Long-Term Outcome. Together with his father, the late academician Evgeny Demidchik, he played a central role in establishing justified approaches to the treatment of childhood thyroid cancer and analyzing the results of therapy after chernobyl. Prof. Ilya Likhtarev, coauthor of Chapter 8, Thyroid Cancer Risk in Ukraine Following the Chernobyl Accident

(The Ukrainian–American Cohort Thyroid Study), was responsible for calculating the doses to those affected by the Chernobyl accident. Our sincere condolences go to their families; they will be sadly missed by the global thyroid and radiation communities.

ACKNOWLEDGMENTS

We gratefully acknowledge the Nippon Foundation and the Sasakawa Memorial Health Foundation for their long-standing support from Chernobyl to Fukushima.

REFERENCES

Ando, R., 2016. Reclaiming our lives in the wake of a nuclear plant accident. Clin. Oncol. (R Coll. Radiol.) 28 (4), 275e276.

Committee to Assess Health Risks from Exposure to Low Levels of Ionizing Radiation. Health risks from exposure to low levels of Ionizing Radiation: BEIR VII phase 2. Washington, DC: National Academy Press; 2006.

Dean, D.S., Gharib, H., 2008. Epidemiology of thyroid nodules. Best Pract. Res. Clin. Endocrinol. Metabol. 22 (6), 901−911.

Hasegawa, A., Ohira, T., Maeda, M., Yasumura, S., Tanigawa, K., 2016. Emergency responses and health consequences after the Fukushima accident; evacuation and relocation. Clin. Oncol. (R Coll. Radiol.) 28 (4), 237e244.

Hawton, K., Bergen, H., Simkin, S., Arensman, E., Corcoran, P., Cooper, J., et al., 2011. Impact of different pack sizes of paracetamol in the United Kingdom and Ireland on intentional overdoses: a comparative study. BMC Public Health 11, 460.

Hendry, J.H., Simon, S.L., Wojcik, A., Sohrabi, M., Burkart, W., Cardis, E., et al., 2009. Human exposure to high natural background radiation: what can it teach us about radiation risks? J. Radiol. Protect. 29 (0), A29−A42.

IAEA report, 2015. The Fukushima Dai-ichi accident 2015. Technical Volume 4/5. Available at: http://www-pub.iaea.org/MTCD/Publications/PDF/AdditionalVolumes/P1710/Pub1710-TV4-Web.pdf.

Kim, E., Kurihara, O., Kunishima, N., Momose, T., Ishikawa, T., Akashi, M., 2016. Internal thyroid doses to Fukushima residents − estimateon and issues remaining. J. Rad. Res. 57 (S1), i118−i126.

Saenko, V.A., Thomas, G.A., Yamashita, S., 2017. Meeting report: the fifth international expert symposium in Fukushima on radiation and health. Environ. Health 16, 3.

UNSCEAR report, 2013. Levels and effects of radiation exposure due to the nuclear accident after the 2011 great east-Japan earthquake and tsunami, Volume 1, Annex A. Available at: http://www.unscear.org/docs/reports/2013/1406336_Report_2013_Annex_A_Ebook_website.pdf.

UNSCEAR Report to the General Assembly of the United Nations, 2008. Annex D. Health effects due to radiation from the Chernobyl accident. Available at: http://www.unscear.org/docs/reports/2008/Advance_copy_Annex_D_Chernobyl_Report.pdf.

WHO report on health risk assessment from the nuclear accident after the 2011 Great East Japan earthquake and tsunami, based on a preliminary dose estimation 2013. Available at:http://apps.who.int/iris/bitstream/10665/78218/1/9789241505130_eng.pdf?ua.1.

Yasumura, S., Hosoya, M., Yamashita, S., Kamiya, K., Abe, M., Akashi, M., et al., 2012. Study protocol for the Fukushima Health Management Survey. J. Epidemiol. 22 (5), 375−383.

PART I

Overview: Keynote Lectures

CHAPTER *1*

Thirty Years After Chernobyl—Overview of the Risks of Thyroid Cancer, Based Upon the UNSCEAR Scientific Reports (2008–2012)

Wolfgang Weiss
Federal Office for Radiation Protection, Emmendingen, Germany

INTRODUCTION

Thyroid cancer is one of the least frequent causes of death from cancer but one of the most important radiation-induced malignancies during a nuclear accident with off-site radiological consequences. In the early phase of such an accident, there is a significant potential for thyroid cancer induction resulting not only from external radiation exposure, but also from internal exposure due to inhalation and ingestion of milk products and food. Before the Chernobyl accident, most of the knowledge on thyroid cancer risk in humans was related to external exposures.

One aim of the thyroid screening programs initiated after a nuclear accident is the timely identification of members of the population with a sufficient level of thyroid exposure as a basis for subsequent medical check-up. The available evidence shows that earlier diagnoses will result in reduced morbidity and mortality. In addition, reliable information about thyroid exposures can be used as the basis for planning longer-term medical services, for prognoses of the health consequences of the exposures incurred, for the design of epidemiological studies, as well as for reassurance measures.

DOSE AND RISK ASSESSMENT METHODOLOGIES

After the Chernobyl accident the assessment of radiation-induced thyroid cancer risk was based on in vivo measurements of the thyroid dose and observations of the incidence of thyroid cancer based on mass screening programs.

Thyroid Cancer and Nuclear Accidents. DOI: http://dx.doi.org/10.1016/B978-0-12-812768-1.00001-0

The contamination of fresh milk with ^{131}I and the lack of prompt and effective countermeasures resulted in high organ doses of the thyroid. The contributions of short-lived radionuclides as compared to the doses resulting from ^{131}I ranged from 0.003 to 0.1, with median values of approximately 0.02 for both cases and controls (Gavrilin et al., 2004). The contribution of external exposures to the thyroid was also very low.

The assessment of the ^{131}I thyroid content was in many cases based on in vivo measurements of the gamma dose rate. It included the measurement of the background dose rate as well as the contribution of extrathyroid radiation from other radionuclides distributed inside and on the surface of the human body. The extrathyroid radiation was recorded simultaneously with the radiation of ^{131}I in the thyroid. Ignoring extrathyroid radiation can result in an overestimation of the ^{131}I content in the thyroid by a factor of up to 3–4 (Zvonova, 2000).

The choice of the ^{131}I intake function into the human body is a critical parameter for the assessment of the organ dose. It was in many cases based on the results of repeated gamma dose rate measurements for individuals over time. The analysis of the variation of the measured dose rates of an individual with time is a very promising way to achieve high-quality thyroid dose estimates. The observed reduction of the ^{131}I content in the thyroid is characterized by a half-life of about 8 days (Bratilova et al., 2003).

The calculation of the thyroid dose was based on state-of-the-art biokinetic and dosimetric models (Balonov et al., 2000). Additional information was obtained from regular screening cycles (Stezhko et al., 2004; Zablotska et al., 2010; Brenner et al., 2011) and sampling of thyroid cancer tissue. Important sources of uncertainty in the calculation of internal exposures are measurement uncertainties (measurement geometry, energy range, spectrum of the background radiation, mass as well as dimensions of the measured person), the time and route of intake, the nuclide composition of the incorporated material and the uncertainties of parameters of the biokinetic and dosimetric models. Various methods have been used to quantify and minimize the uncertainties at each stage of the dose calculations. Annex B of the 2012 UNSCEAR report provides a detailed scientific discussion of the relevant methodologies as well as the current knowledge in this field.

EVIDENCE ON THYROID EXPOSURE AND CANCER RISK AFTER THE CHERNOBYL ACCIDENT

The total number of direct thyroid measurements for children in Ukraine, Belarus, and the Russian Federation reported in the scientific literature to date is about 160,000. Individual dose assessments are available for about 27,000 children covering a range of the mean thyroid dose from well below 0.1 Gy to about 60 Gy (Gavrilin et al., 1999).

Most of the available evidence about thyroid cancer incidence among those in Belarus and Ukraine, who were exposed during childhood or adolescence, is based on results of epidemiological studies. The study results show trends of increased frequency of the cancer incidence with absorbed dose to the thyroid primarily from internal exposure. Significant differences in thyroid cancer incidence related to age and gender of the children were observed. The observed increase of thyroid cancer incidence was primarily among the children under age 10 years at the time of the accident. For those born after 1986, there was no evidence for such an increase. The baseline cancer incidence among males who were 10 years old at the time of the accident was found to be more than a factor of four lower than among females. A minimum latency period for the identification of radiation-induced childhood thyroid cancer was found to be 4−5 years. By 1995, the incidence of childhood thyroid cancer related to the Chernobyl accident increased to four cases per 100,000 per year as compared to 0.03−0.05 cases per 100,000 per year prior to the accident (UNSCEAR, 2008).

The key question remains whether the observed increase in thyroid cancer frequency in the population and in individuals can indeed be attributed to radiation exposure from the accident (UNSCEAR, 2012). The available evidence remains somewhat uncertain. The main reasons are the lack of conceptual clarity of the results of ultrasonography and mass screening techniques in terms of future cancer development. Strong indication that the increased use of the applied screening methodologies was not the main reason for the higher observed frequency of thyroid cancer is obtained from studies of those born after 1986, which showed no evidence for an increase in the frequency of thyroid cancer. On the other hand, medical surveillance among this group or iodine insufficiency cannot be ruled out completely as confounding factors; iodine insufficiency could have influenced the thyroid cancer risks both by affecting the uptake of radioiodines at the time of exposure and altering the thyroid function following the exposure (Kanno et al., 1992; Tronko et al., 2005). In the absence of a biomarker to distinguish a radiation-related thyroid cancer from one that occurs due to other causes, an observed thyroid cancer in an individual among the population of those exposed as children or adolescents at the time of the accident cannot be unequivocally attributed to the radiation exposure after the accident. Nevertheless the available evidence strongly supports the conclusion that the observed increase of the frequency of the thyroid cancer risk can, at least in part, be attributed to internal exposure due to ^{131}I from the Chernobyl accident. It has been estimated by UNSCEAR (2008, 2012) that about 60% of the Belarusian thyroid cancer cases and 30% of the Ukrainian cases among those who were children or adolescents at the time of the accident may be related to radiation exposure (Jacob et al., 2006).

The increase in thyroid cancer incidence observed among those exposed as children or adolescents in Belarus, the Russian Federation, and Ukraine showed no signs of diminishing up to 20 years after exposure. Although thyroid cancer incidence continued to increase for this group, up to 2005 only 15 cases had proved fatal. The total number of thyroid cancer cases registered between 1991 and 2015 in those who were under 18 in 1986, and resided in the whole of Belarus, the northwestern oblasts of Ukraine, and the four Russian regions continued to rise to reach a total of more than about 16,000 in 2015 (Drozdovitch et al., 2015; Likhtarov et al., 2014; UNSCEAR, 2010). This number is about a factor of 2.5 larger than the number of thyroid cancer cases registered in the same cohort during the period 1991–2005. No analysis is available at this time which fraction of this number can be attributed to radiation. The UNSCEAR Committee requested the secretariat to prepare a short paper on the evaluation of thyroid cancer data in regions affected by the Chernobyl accident, with a view to discussion and acceptance at the 64th session of the Committee in 2017.

DISCUSSION

Different detector types and calibration factors have been used for dose rate measurements. There is a need for harmonization to reduce the inherent assessment uncertainties. This could be achieved by verification measurements including measurements of an unknown activity of mock iodine circulated as part of emergency preparedness measures (trills and exercises). The calibration procedures have to take into account the age of the screened persons: children, adolescents, and adults. The identification of a relevant thyroid dose in young children requires MDAs of the detectors used as low as 10−20 mGy.

There are two key factors that influenced the conclusive identification of a radiation-induced increase of the incidence of thyroid cancer, i.e., the latency period for the development of thyroid cancer and the screening effect. The analyses by UNSCEAR (2012) demonstrate that an absorbed dose to the thyroid between >100 and 250 mGy may result in a measurable increase of thyroid cancer development in children exposed at ages of between 0 and 18 years. Younger ages have a higher probability to develop a thyroid cancer and a lower spontaneous incidence rate. The ability to attribute an increase in a population to radiation exposure is higher for infants than for adolescents.

A substantial increase of the incidence of thyroid cancer has been observed through mass screening programs during the past decade in high-income countries (Vaccarella et al., 2016). This increase was caused by the identification of intrathyroidal papillary thyroid microcarcinomas, i.e., abnormalities that meet the pathologic definition of cancer but may never progress to cause symptoms or death during a patient's lifetime. This type of increasing diagnosis has led to concerns about "over"diagnosis as a result of mass screening programs because "over"diagnosed patients do not have benefit from the detection and treatment of their "cancer," they can only be harmed. According to IARC (2016) the "over"diagnosis of tumors must be considered as a major confounding factor for the assessment of thyroid cancer risk.

CONCLUSION

One of the big challenges during the early response to a nuclear accident with off-site consequences is the question whether screening programs will produce more benefits for the affected population than potential harm (unjustified invasive interventions, psychological stress, ethical considerations, stigmatization, social impact). The availability of reliable exposure assessment methodologies has been and remains a key prerequisite to minimize the inherent uncertainties in decision-making.

The lack of common protocols for measurement and for recording the information about the screened persons as well as for the assessment of the relevant exposure pathways (ingestion, inhalation, physical and chemical forms of the radioiodines) can result in substantial uncertainties in interpreting the measurement results. Basic concept and methodologies (prognostic transport models, real-time environmental measurement systems, basic assessment methodologies) have to be developed further and trained during preparedness as a basis for a realistic characterization of representative groups of the affected population (number of people, age spectrum, expected dose range, age-dependent detection limits). Proposals are available in the scientific literature for state-of-the-art methodological approaches, which can be considered to represent good practice. They include the application of standardized, harmonized, and calibrated equipment of sufficient detection capability (MDA), standardized (age-dependent) detector calibration methodologies, common protocols for measurement performance and registration of the results, availability of trained personal, as well as agreed communication concepts. What remains to be done is the implementation of these methodologies in the operational world.

Despite all the valuable evidence derived after the Chernobyl accident there are key scientific questions to be resolved through future research. These include the continuing need to quantify the thyroid cancer risk for young children at organ doses below 100 mGy, the thyroid cancer risk for adults at low doses, as well as the improvement of the scientific basis for the attribution of radiation-induced thyroid risks of infants, children, and adults. This would require improved understanding of the effects of confounding factors like the influence of iodine deficiency on thyroid cancer risk on thyroid cancer development as well as the effect of "over"diagnosis of mass screening programs. The identification of relevant markers of individual sensitivity as well as markers of epigenetic effects remains a challenge for scientific research.

Based on the lessons learned from Chernobyl, there are many opportunities to improve the preparedness for and the response to any future accident and to reduce the existing uncertainties of thyroid dose and risk assessments by agreement on

• standardized, harmonized, and calibrated equipment of sufficient detection capability (MDA);

- standardized (age-dependent) detector calibration methodologies;
- common protocols for measurement performance and registration of the results;
- standardized and harmonized methodologies for mass screening and long-term follow-up.

It is highly recommended to use these lessons learned and to implement appropriate arrangements in the operational world.

REFERENCES

Balonov, M.I., et al., 2000. Methodology of internal dose reconstruction for a Russian population after the Chernobyl accident. Radiat. Prot. Dosim. 92 (1–3), 247–253.

Bratilova, A., et al., 2003. ^{131}I content in the human throid estimated from direct measurements of the inhabitants of Russian areas contaminated due to the Chernobyl accicent. Radiat. Prot. Dosim. 105 (1–4), 623–626.

Brenner, A.V., Tronko, M.D., Hatch, M., Bogdanova, T.I., Oliynik, V.A., Lubin, J.H., et al., 2011. I-131 dose response for incident thyroid cancers in Ukraine related to the Chornobyl accident. Environ. Health Perspect. 119, 933–939.

Drozdovitch, V., Minenko, V., Golovanov, I., 2015. Thyroid dose estimates for a cohort of Belarusian children exposed to ^{131}I from the Chernobyl accident: assessment of uncertainties. Radiat. Res. 184 (2), 203–218.

Gavrilin, Y., et al., 1999. Chernobyl accident: reconstruction of thyroid dose for inhabitants of the Republic of Belarus. Health Phys. 76, 105–119.

Gavrilin, Y., et al., 2004. Case-control study of Chernobyl-related thyroid cancer among children of Belarus. Part I: estimation of individual thyroid doses resulting from intakes of ^{131}I, short-lived radioiodines (^{132}I, ^{133}I, ^{135}I), and short-lived radiotelluriums (^{131m}Te and ^{132}Te). Health Phys. 86, 565–585.

IARC (2016) Overdiagnosis is a major driver of the thyroid cancer epidemic: up to 50–90% of thyroid cancers in women in high-income countries estimated to be overdiagnoses, press release No. 246.

Jacob, P., et al., 2006. Thyroid cancer among Ukrainians and Belarusians who were children or adolescents at the time of the Chernobyl accident. J. Radiol. Prot. 26 (1), 51–67.

Kanno, J., et al., 1992. Tumor-promoting effects of both iodine deficiency and iodine excess in the rat thyroid. Toxicol. Pathol. 20, 226–235.

Likhtarov, I., et al., 2014. Thyroid cancer study among Ukrainian children exposed to radiation after the Chornbyl accident: improved estimates of the thyroid doses to the cohort members. Health Phys. 106 (3), 370–396.

Stezhko, V.A., Buglova, E.E., Danilova, L.A., et al., 2004. A cohort study of thyroid cancer and other thyroid diseases after the Chernobyl accident: design and methods. Radiat. Res. 161 (4), 481–492.

Tronko, M., et al., 2005. Iodine excretion in regions of Ukraine affected by iodine excretion in regions of Ukraine affected by the Chornobyl accident: experience of the Ukrainian-American cohort study of thyroid cancer and other thyroid diseases. Thyroid 15 (11), 1291–1297.

UNSCEAR (2008) Sources and Effects of Ionizing Radiation. Volume II: Effects. Scientific Annexes C, D and E. UNSCEAR 2008 Report. United Nations Scientific Committee on the Effects of Atomic Radiation. United Nations Sales Publication E.11.IX.3, United Nations, New York, 2011.

UNSCEAR, 2010. Summary of Low-dose Radiation Effects on Health. United Nations, New York.

UNSCEAR (2012) Sources, Effects and Risks of Ionizing Radiation. Volume II: Scientific Annex B. UNSCEAR Report 2012. United Nations Sales Publication E.16.IX.1, United Nations, New York, 2015.

Vaccarella, S., et al., 2016. Worldwide Thyroid-Cancer Epidemic? The Increasing Impact of Overdiagnosis. N. Engl. J. Med. 375, 7.

Zablotska, L.B., Ron, E., Rozhko, A.V., Hatch, M., Polyanskaya, O.N., Brenner, A.V., et al., 2010. Thyroid cancer risk in Belarus among children and adolescents exposed to radioiodine after the Chornobyl accident. Br. J. Cancer. 104 (1), 181.

Zvonova, I., 2000. Mass internal exposure monitoring of the population in Russia after the Chernobyl accident. Radiat. Prot. Dosim. 89 (3–4), 173–178.

FURTHER READING

Drozdovitch, V., et al., 2013. Thyroid dose estimates for a cohort of Belarusian children exposed to radiation from the Chernobyl accident. Radiat. Res. 179 (5), 597–609.

Zvonova, I.A., Balonov, M.I., Bratilova, A.A., 1998. Thyroid dose reconstruction for the population of Russia after the Chernobyl accident. Radiat. Prot. Dosim. 79 (1–4), 175–178.

CHAPTER 2

Thirty Years After the Chernobyl Nuclear Power Plant Accident: Contribution From Japan—"Confirming the Increase of Childhood Thyroid Cancer"

Shigenobu Nagataki and Shunichi Yamashita
Nagasaki University, Nagasaki, Japan

THE INITIAL CIRCUMSTANCES OF THE CHERNOBYL NPP ACCIDENT

The Chernobyl nuclear power plant (NPP) accident, the worst in the history of mankind, occurred during the Cold War era, and information released from the USSR about it was extremely limited from 1986 to 1990. In 1990, the Soviet government made a formal request to the International Atomic Energy Agency (IAEA) for a study on the radiation effects and began accepting investigations from foreign countries. The Japanese government implemented a collaborative project for the Japan—USSR specialists through the Ministry of Foreign Affairs along with financial cooperation from the World Health Organization (WHO)'s preliminary research project on health consequences. The Nippon Foundation, in response to the direct request from the Soviet government, dispatched a research team of Japanese specialists to the site in 1990 through the Sasakawa Memorial Health Foundation, which later became the origins of the Chernobyl Sasakawa Health and Medical Cooperation Project.

The Chernobyl Sasakawa Health and Medical Cooperation Project began with a presentation ceremony of medical examination vehicles on April 26, 1991 in Moscow's Red Square. The objective was to conduct health screenings for thyroid cancer and leukemia among children who were aged 0—10 years at the time of the accident. To be more precise, the project began with the training and creation of examination protocol at the Medical Radiological Research

Thyroid Cancer and Nuclear Accidents. DOI: http://dx.doi.org/10.1016/B978-0-12-812768-1.00002-2

Center in Obninsk on May 1st of that year. Five mobile diagnostic buses loaded with ultrasonic thyroid examination devices, blood analysis machines, and whole-body counters to measure internal radiation exposure were donated by Japan; the screening project began in five diagnostic centers arranged for by the Soviet side in the area around Chernobyl. Specialists dispatched from Nagasaki University, Hiroshima University, and Radiation Effects Research Foundation were the principal persons involved, and they played a central role in the training and implementation of concrete examination at the five centers.

As a result of the project, 160,000 screenings were completed over a 5-year period in children aged 0–10 years at the time of the accident. Blood samples were also taken from all subjects and an analysis was done on the whole blood count (WBC) and blood cell pictures. The levels of thyroid hormones (TSH and T4) and autoantibodies against the thyroid were measured in all subjects. The first 3-year results of thyroid examination were reported for the first time during the Nagasaki symposium on Chernobyl (Yamashita et al., 1994). Beginning a few years after the accident, urine samples were also taken in each location to measure the iodine levels, and 5-year data through 1996 were compiled and analyzed (Ashizawa et al., 1997; Yamashita and Shibata, 1997). In addition, comparative studies on the frequency of thyroid cancer among children born before and after the accident and so on were performed (Shibata et al., 2001), resulting in a grand total of screening data for 200,000 individuals collected over the 10-year period.

The full-scale investigative study on health effects of the Chernobyl disaster was implemented on a global scale exactly 20 years before the Fukushima NPP accident and, moreover, was the sole project based on a unified diagnostic standard in the three countries around Chernobyl (Belarus, Ukraine, and Russia). Due to this study, the importance of quality control for diagnostic equipment, unification of diagnostic standards, and the dissemination of accumulated information was fully recognized. In truth, an important contribution to this project was the training of personnel in the affected areas, the mentality for which has been inherited from the Nagasaki Association for Hibakushas' Medical Care (NASHIM). Except for the increase in thyroid cancer among children and adolescents, data, which infer a causal relationship with radiation, were not obtained through the results of this study. In particular, an increase in leukemia or other diseases was not identified. For this reason, the Sasakawa Memorial Health Foundation has provided financial support since 2000 for an international joint research project with the International Agency for Research on Cancer (IARC), which carried out a radiation epidemiology case-control study focusing solely on thyroid cancer among children and adolescents (Cardis et al., 2005).

THE ERA OF ANALYZING AUTHENTICITY AND CAUSE OF INCREASED CHILDHOOD THYROID CANCER AROUND CHERNOBYL

Oral Presentations

In 1991, Professor E.P. Demidchik, the Director of Thyroid Cancer Center in Minsk, Belarus, visited Japan through the Ministry of Foreign Affairs' Japan–USSR bilateral Chernobyl specialists' project and disclosed in Nagasaki that instances of surgery for thyroid cancer at his research center had increased following the accident. It was the first time that this was stated in a country outside of the Soviet Union. However, the results of the IAEA study which had just been published at that time showed that there was no evidence of any health consequences of the accident, and the claim was not discussed much at the press conference thereafter.

Publications

In September, 1992 in the issue of the journal *Nature*, an article was published on the increase in cases of thyroid cancer in Chernobyl, listing among the authors first the Belarus Minister of Health and the directors of Minsk Thyroid Cancer Center and Radiation Medicine Institute (Kazakov et al., 1992). Supporting papers were published consecutively by, amongst others, scientists based at the WHO European Regional Office, Cambridge University, and the University of Pisa faculty. However, objections from others, based at the Japanese Radiation Effects Research Foundation, Oxford University, and the University of Chicago stated that it was too soon to come to the conclusion that "this was caused by radiation" were published as comments to *Nature* at the same time.

Clinical Examination of Childhood Thyroid Cancer Patients

Exchange of ideas and information with experts around the world also began at this time, and the day after the article appeared, 12 experts on thyroid diseases from the USA, various European countries, and Japan, including the author, met in Minsk Cancer Research Institute. As a host, Professor Demidchik introduced the case studies of what seemed to be one patient after the next, their medical histories, surgical records, even displaying pathological specimens, so everyone in attendance concurred on the first day that there was a sizeable number of childhood thyroid cancer patients. The far greater number of childhood thyroid cancer patients than expected was shocking because we, thyroid experts, had never before examined so many young patients at one time. The histopathological diagnosis was papillary thyroid carcinoma in all childhood cases, and although this type of adult cancer usually does not metastasize anywhere except for the cervical lymph nodes, there were many cases of lung metastases. Opinions were divided; those who agreed that the Chernobyl NPP accident was the likely cause of the increase in cases of thyroid cancer in children were mainly the European researchers, whilst the academics based in Japan and America argued that epidemiological studies had not yet been appropriately undertaken and that no conclusion was therefore possible.

International Debates Surrounding Thyroid Cancer

In the period up to 1996, international conferences were frequently held around this issue in various countries around the world, as well as those hosted by the international organizations. As for the author himself, there were three international meetings held in the city of Nagasaki at that time period. Many scholars from different parts of the world debated the topic seriously, and the focus of the discussion was always whether exposure to radiation causes thyroid cancer, or whether the increased frequency was attributable to the Chernobyl NPP accident or not. While a variety of interpretations emerged, the participants consistently evaluated and discussed the evidence in a scientific manner. In particular, there was an argument that without denominator data on the general population, there is no epidemiology, and from that standpoint, the explanation of the increase in thyroid cancer was insufficient on an epidemiological level because even when the number of patients is increased, there is no denominator in terms of background incidence. Later, when denominator data became available, the argument, mainly developed in Russia, was that the number of patients had increased because of the screenings. At an international symposium held in Nagasaki in 1994 (8 years after the accident), academics from the regions around the world that had experienced exposure to radiation (the atomic bomb detonations in Japan, the Marshall Islands, the Hanford nuclear facility in the USA, the Ural Mountains nuclear disaster at Mayak, and the three countries relevant to Chernobyl) as well as representatives from the international authorities such as the WHO, held a public debate, and when at the end, the author, who was acting as the host and moderator, asked the participants to choose between "the increase in thyroid cancer is caused by the Chernobyl disaster" and "it cannot be confirmed at this time; further research into other causes is necessary," all 11 of the presenters voted for further research being needed (Nagataki and Yamashita, 1996). This was the global situation from 1992 to 1995.

International Conference Confirms Increase of Thyroid Cancer

At the time, it was common for international scientists to debate using actual study results, rather than the evaluation of published papers. In 1996, which marked 10 years after the accident, the WHO, European Community (EC), and IAEA hosted a series of international conferences. At a meeting in the first WHO conference, Russian scientists, who had claimed until then that there had been no increase in thyroid cancer, suddenly commented that it was increasing in Russia, just as it was in Belarus and Ukraine. The screenings did have an impact, but when looking at the results for children under age 14 who had been examined using the same methodology every year until 1994, they came to the conclusion that there had been an increase.

The IAEA, WHO, and EC Joint Session where an Increase in Thyroid Cancer and its Cause was Confirmed: "One Decade After Chernobyl"

As the last international conference on the 10th anniversary of the disaster, an international symposium called "One Decade after Chernobyl" was held in Vienna as a joint session of the IAEA, WHO, and EC. The six copresenters (from the UK, the USA, Japan, Russia, Belarus, and Ukraine) held a meeting in advance of the symposium, where Professor E.D. Williams of Cambridge University gave a presentation as the representative speaker, and all six members took the stage during the question and answer time. To summarize the announcements made with regard to the increase in the frequency of thyroid cancer, as people were examined using the same procedure, the impact of the screening would be the same and so it could be said that the number of patients discovered every year who are children under the age of 14 under that system was increasing (One Decade after Chernobyl: Summing up the Consequences of the Accident, 1996). On an epidemiological level, the denominator data would be the number of children in a given country, with the numerator being the study results of the number of children who had surgical operation for thyroid cancer in that year, and so it was reported that "there was an increase in thyroid cancer among children which was caused by the Chernobyl NPP accident." In the debate that followed the presentation, a specialist from the US asked whether there was a relationship with the exposure dose (radiation dose correlation). The answer I remember well, as I was the one who replied, was that, at that time, the relationship between thyroid cancer and dose to which that patient had been exposed had not been investigated. In actuality, after the accident the radioiodine-131 in the thyroid gland was measured in more than 100,000 children, but there was no reliable measured value, which could be used epidemiologically as the exposure dose, and so at that time the relationship between dose and thyroid cancer incidence was not understood. Even so, the reason for coming to the conclusion that "there was an increase in childhood thyroid cancer caused by the Chernobyl NPP accident" was described as the existence of strong circumstantial evidence, both chronological (a clear increase since 1991) and geographical (the three nations all being exposed to radiation fallout). The first case-control study on thyroid cancer in the children of Belarus was published in 1998, suggesting a relationship between thyroid cancer in children and estimated radiation dose from the Chernobyl accident (Astakhova et al., 1998).

Thyroid Cancer in Children Born After the Accident in Belarus

After this, independent of the movements of international organizations, ultrasound examinations were carried out using the same procedure from 1996 to 2001 through the Chernobyl Sasakawa Health and Medical Cooperation Project in the city of Gomel, which was the region of Belarus with the highest frequency of thyroid cancer, on children born after the accident who did not have internal exposure to radioiodine. This study has proved that compared with children born before the accident, children born after had no increase in thyroid cancer whatsoever, leading to the presumption that the increase in thyroid cancer had indeed been caused by the Chernobyl NPP accident (Shibata et al., 2001). These results were a major achievement for the Japanese team. Moreover, the outcome of a case-control investigation conducted in a collaboration with the IARC clarified that the risk of thyroid cancer was dependent on the dose of radioiodine exposure to the thyroid gland (Cardis et al., 2005).

International Conferences on the 20th Anniversary

With regard to thyroid cancer, the research results on subsequent variations in the frequency of occurrence are important. Data on the number of thyroid cancer surgeries in Belarus, which were reported at the time, provided valuable information through the annual shifts in the age breakdown at the time of surgery. From 1986 to 1988, the frequency of thyroid cancer among children was approximately one or two out of a million, but this gradually increased to as much as 40 per million in 1995, declining thereafter until reaching nearly the same level as it had been prior to the accident in 2002. Correspondingly, the age group with the highest number of thyroid cancer surgeries shifted over to adolescents, with the long-term risk of developing thyroid malignancy inferred to be concentrated in children who were aged 0–10 years at the time of exposure (Demidchik et al., 2007).

Results of the Study on Dose–Response Relationship of Thyroid Cancer

Although the correlation of the level of radiation dose with thyroid cancer was not accepted at the international conference held on the 10th year after the disaster, 15 years later bilateral America–Belarus and America–Ukraine projects were able to successfully reconstruct the complicated respective radiation doses (albeit with the weak point of not being a direct measurement) and announced that there was a significant correlation (Brenner et al., 2011; Zablotska et al., 2011). In both studies, the internal exposure dose through the oral ingestion of food contaminated by the initial fallout of radioiodine (primarily contaminated milk) was identified as a significant contributor to the thyroid dose.

Treatment Results in Thyroid Cancer Patients

The UNSCEAR report on the 25th year since the accident announced that 6000 people had been diagnosed for thyroid cancer, but recorded that 15 had died (UNSCEAR 2008 Report to the General Assembly with Scientific Annexes, 2011). With the astounding achievement of a 99.75% survival rate, treatment results were reported on as follows.

In a follow-up examination of 740 patients in Belarus, the survival rates after 5 years and then after 10 years were 99.7% and 99.2%, respectively (Demidchik et al., 2006). A total of 234 Belarussian children were treated with radioiodine-131 in Germany, and in follow-up surveys conducted 11.3 years later (not the average time, but the median), one child was reported to have died (Reiners et al., 2013). Seventy percent of thyroid cancers were also reported to be under 2 cm in size. A survival rate of 99% even after cancer diagnosis, completely unlike other forms of human cancer, is something that we must take particular note of. Similar prognosis analysis was reported in patients from Russia (Rumyantsev et al., 2011).

THE FUKUSHIMA HEALTH MANAGEMENT SURVEY WITH REGARD TO THYROID ULTRASOUND EXAMINATIONS

Thyroid ultrasound examinations for all children registered in Fukushima prefecture are currently in progress under the established diagnostic protocol (Suzuki et al., 2016). In cases where thyroid cancer is diagnosed, medical treatment is carried out according to the recommendation of a thyroid expert. However, the parents in Fukushima remain concerned that their child might develop thyroid cancer in the future, despite being informed that their child's test found no abnormalities at that time. These are the real difficulties with examinations after the NPP accident, and the decisions based on scientific knowledge are required to give reassurance to worried parents. It is now clear that the Fukushima accident is substantially different from Chernobyl in respect of the thyroid radiation dose (Nagataki and Takamura, 2016). However, a research survey conducted over a long period of time and the verification of its validity are always indispensable. For this very reason, it is vital to gather the world's wisdom when holding the 5th International Expert Symposium in Fukushima on Radiation and Health.

After the Fukushima NPP accident, medical personnel throughout Japan with specialist licenses of the Japan Thyroid Association and other related organizations for ultrasound examination worked together to develop a state-of-the-art thyroid ultrasound examination protocol using the latest medical instruments and most uptodate knowledge that would be appropriate for use, even in the case of repeated occurrences of thyroid cancer following rounds of screening as there were after Chernobyl. However, conducting such a sensitive screening procedure is not without risks. There is always the possibility of overdiagnosis and therefore unnecessary medical treatment, which poses its own risks. For this reason there is also a need to minimize every aspect of the potential risks associated with thyroid screening among the population of Fukushima (Nagataki, 2016). It is therefore necessary that academicians and experts from Japan and from around the world continue to discuss the matter thoroughly and to analyze the situation in order to derive policies to address these issues. This will continue to be important in allaying the remaining fears of the local population in Fukushima.

SUMMARY

This chapter has discussed the Japanese contribution to "Confirming the Increase of Childhood Thyroid Cancer" after the Chernobyl NPP accident. One of the lessons learned from Chernobyl is not only the difficulty of confirmation of the cause-and-effect relationship between radiation exposure and thyroid cancer risk but also how to understand and implement health monitoring, especially with respect to thyroid ultrasound examination, of the affected population over a long time period. Having faced an NPP accident, it is my most sincere hope that the residents of Fukushima, having to live with the anxiety of the possibility of needing to undergo thyroid ultrasound examinations and the possibility of developing cancer in the future, gain a fuller understanding of health and the natural history of abnormal thyroid findings, including cancer. Living with an uncertain future, it is essential that they keep hope alive while taking steps along the path to reconstruction and recovery.

REFERENCES

Ashizawa, K., Shibata, Y., Yamashita, S., Namba, H., Hoshi, M., Yokoyama, N., et al., 1997. Prevalence of goiter and urinary iodine excretion levels in children around Chernobyl. J. Clin. Endocrinol. Metab. 82 (10), 3430–3433. Available from: http://dx.doi.org/10.1210/jcem.82.10.4285.

Astakhova, L.N., Anspaugh, L.R., Beebe, G.W., Bouville, A., Drozdovitch, V.V., Garber, V., et al., 1998. Chernobyl-related thyroid cancer in children of Belarus: a case-control study. Radiat. Res. 150 (3), 349–356.

Brenner, A.V., Tronko, M.D., Hatch, M., Bogdanova, T.I., Oliynik, V.A., Lubin, J.H., et al., 2011. I-131 dose response for incident thyroid cancers in Ukraine related to the Chornobyl accident. Environ. Health Perspect. 119 (7), 933–939. Available from: http://dx.doi.org/10.1289/ehp.1002674.

Cardis, E., Kesminiene, A., Ivanov, V., Malakhova, I., Shibata, Y., Khrouch, V., et al., 2005. Risk of thyroid cancer after exposure to 131I in childhood. J. Natl. Cancer Inst. 97 (10), 724–732. Available from: http://dx.doi.org/10.1093/jnci/dji129.

Demidchik, Y.E., Demidchik, E.P., Reiners, C., Biko, J., Mine, M., Saenko, V.A., et al., 2006. Comprehensive clinical assessment of 740 cases of surgically treated thyroid cancer in children of Belarus. Ann. Surg. 243 (4), 525–532. Available from: http://dx.doi.org/10.1097/01.sla.0000205977.74806.0b.

Demidchik, Y.E., Saenko, V.A., Yamashita, S., 2007. Childhood thyroid cancer in Belarus, Russia, and Ukraine after Chernobyl and at present. Arq. Bras. Endocrinol. Metab. 51 (5), 748–762.

Kazakov, V.S., Demidchik, E.P., Astakhova, L.N., 1992. Thyroid cancer after Chernobyl. Nature 359 (6390), 21. Available from: http://dx.doi.org/10.1038/359021a0.

Nagataki, S., 2016. Minimizing the health effects of the nuclear accident in Fukushima on thyroids. Eur. Thyroid J. 5 (4). Available from: http://dx.doi.org/10.1159/000448890.

Nagataki, S., Takamura, N., 2016. Radioactive doses − predicted and actual − and likely health effects. Clin. Oncol. 28 (4), 245–254. Available from: http://dx.doi.org/10.1016/j.clon.2015.12.028.

Nagataki, S., Yamashita, Y. (Eds.), 1996. Nagasaki Symposium on Radiation and Human Health: Proposal from Nagasaki. Elsevier, Amsterdam.

One Decade after Chernobyl: Summing up the Consequences of the Accident, 1996. International Atomic Energy Agency, Vienna.

Reiners, C., Biko, J., Haenscheid, H., Hebestreit, H., Kirinjuk, S., Baranowski, O., et al., 2013. Twenty-five years after Chernobyl: outcome of radioiodine treatment in children and adolescents with very high-risk radiation-induced differentiated thyroid carcinoma. J. Clin. Endocrinol. Metab. 98 (7), 3039–3048. Available from: http://dx.doi.org/10.1210/jc.2013-1059.

Rumyantsev, P.O., Saenko, V.A., Ilyin, A.A., Stepanenko, V.F., Rumyantseva, U.V., Abrosimov, A.Y., et al., 2011. Radiation exposure does not significantly contribute to the risk of recurrence of Chernobyl thyroid cancer. J. Clin. Endocrinol. Metab. 96 (2), 385–393. Available from: http://dx.doi.org/10.1210/jc.2010-1634.

Shibata, Y., Yamashita, S., Masyakin, V.B., Panasyuk, G.D., Nagataki, S., 2001. 15 years after Chernobyl: new evidence of thyroid cancer. Lancet 358 (9297), 1965–1966. http://dx.doi.org/10.1016/S0140-6736(01)06971-9.

Suzuki, S., Yamashita, S., Fukushima, T., Nakano, K., Midorikawa, S., Ohtsuru, A., et al., 2016. The protocol and preliminary baseline survey results of the thyroid ultrasound examination in Fukushima. Endocr. J. 63 (3), 315–321. Available from: http://dx.doi.org/10.1507/endocrj.EJ15-0726.

UNSCEAR 2008 Report to the General Assembly with Scientific Annexes, 2008. Volume II Annex D. Health Effects due to Radiation from the Chernobyl Accident. United Nations, New York.

Yamashita, S., Namba, H., Ito, M., Ashizawa, K., 1994. In: Nagataki, S. (Ed.), Chernobyl Sasakawa Health and Medical Cooperation-1994. Elsevier, Amsterdam-Tokyo.

Yamashita, S., Shibata, Y. (Eds.), 1997. Chernobyl: A Decade. Elsevier, Amsterdam.

Zablotska, L.B., Ron, E., Rozhko, A.V., Hatch, M., Polyanskaya, O.N., Brenner, A.V., et al., 2011. Thyroid cancer risk in Belarus among children and adolescents exposed to radioiodine after the Chornobyl accident. Br. J. Cancer 104 (1), 181–187. Available from: http://dx.doi.org/10.1038/sj.bjc.6605967.

CHAPTER 3

From Chernobyl to Fukushima and Beyond—A Focus on Thyroid Cancer

John D. Boice Jr.[1,2]

[1]National Council on Radiation Protection and Measurements, Bethesda, MD, United States
[2]Vanderbilt University School of Medicine, Nashville, TN, United States

INTRODUCTION

The *1st International Expert Symposium in Fukushima on Radiation and Health* was sponsored by the Nippon Foundation in September 2011, just 6 months after the Great East Japan earthquake, tsunami, and nuclear power plant (NPP) accident (FMU, 2015). The *5th International Expert Symposium in Fukushima on Radiation and Health, Chernobyl + 30, Fukushima + 5—Lessons and Solutions for Fukushima's Thyroid Question* was held in September 2016 (Nippon Foundation, 2016; Boice, 2016). Much has been learned on remediation, stakeholder engagement, resettlement, mental health, mitigation, waste management, communication, environmental monitoring, and health management. It should be stressed that the Fukushima Management team has done a marvelous job these past 5 years in these difficult circumstances, not just with thyroid screenings, pregnancy issues, and mental health concerns, but many other issues of importance to the people of Fukushima have had to be dealt with day and night (Yasumura et al., 2012).

The focus of the 5th symposium was to address the thyroid cancer issues that arose after screening 300,000 children with sophisticated ultrasound equipment (Suzuki et al, 2016; Suzuki, 2016a,b; Normile, 2016; Wakeford, 2016). The survey was initiated to be responsive to public concerns and not for scientific reasons. Lumps and bumps were detected and fine-needle biopsies uncovered thyroid carcinomas and tumors at a high rate. Even though the tumors could not possibly be related to radiation exposure, they nonetheless were real, and public anxiety has increased.

Thyroid Cancer and Nuclear Accidents. DOI: http://dx.doi.org/10.1016/B978-0-12-812768-1.00003-4

This chapter will address briefly a number of important but wide-ranging issues: the radiation doses received by populations living around the Chernobyl and Fukushima reactors, the health effects observed or expected, what is known about radiation-induced thyroid cancer from over 60 years of epidemiologic studies, the difference between surveys and studies (surveys are for people while studies are for science), mental health problems being an immediate- and long-term consequence of the Fukushima accident, and the excess thyroid cancers reported in the screening surveys are an artifact related to the sensitive ultrasound technique used, and not due to radiation.

Foremost it should always be remembered that radiation risk and theoretical projections of risk pale in comparison with the $\sim 20,000$ immediate deaths after the tsunami (including over 1000 children), the destruction of entire villages, and the disruption to hundreds of thousands of lives (ANN, 2012).

Fukushima is not Chernobyl, neither in extent of radiation released nor in health effects (Boice, 2012; Wakeford, 2016; Yamashita et al., 2016). Population doses from the Fukushima reactor accident are tiny and of little health consequence (UNSCEAR, 2014; Kamiya et al., 2016; Tokonami et al., 2012). The fear of radiation has caused immediate and lasting anxiety affecting health (Yoshida et al., 2016a). When modeled doses differ from measured doses (Nagataki et al., 2013), change the model or rely upon measured dose. Do not misuse collective doses (González et al., 2013). It is wrong to multiply a trivial dose times a large population and compute theoretical (and impossible) numbers of future cancers. We know much about radiation-induced thyroid cancer from patients exposed for medical conditions, Chernobyl, and from atomic bomb survivors (Ron et al., 2012; Boice, 2005, 2006). Radiation causes thyroid cancer, but not immediately. Radiation causes thyroid cancer, but not after trivial doses (no theoretical increase is detectable). Radiation causes thyroid cancer, but primarily among those under age 5 years at exposure and not among adults. The screening survey of childhood exposure does not indicate any radiation excess, but an overdiagnosis due to the very sensitive ultrasound technique (Vaccarella et al., 2016). Surveys should never be called studies; the surveys have no ability to find radiation associations even if they exist. Failure to communicate effectively contributed to the epidemic of thyroid cancer after Chernobyl, and the distrust of government after Fukushima, and raised anxiety among people. Mental health issues remain a serious current effect of the anxiety raised from the accident, and resources should be committed for treatment (Yoshida et al., 2016a). Japan as well as the world needs to find and train radiation professionals to handle current needs as well as future needs. Engage with stakeholders at all times (Nagataki and Takamura, 2016). Again, remember that these surveys are not for science but for the people (thanks to Mr. Tanami for the clarity of this distinction between surveys and studies).

FUKUSHIMA IS NOT CHERNOBYL

Fukushima is not Chernobyl in terms of radiation releases and in terms of the potential for health effects (Wakeford, 2016; Yamashita et al., 2016; Boice, 2012). While the Japanese government lost credibility because of the failure to communicate effectively, they did most things right. There was sheltering in place, evacuation, and restriction of the food supply. In contrast, after Chernobyl there was little immediate action and the drinking of contaminated milk by children resulted in an epidemic of thyroid cancers. This will not be the case following Fukushima. The population doses were very low and the pathway from ingesting large quantities of milk or contaminated food was restricted. Doses were mainly from inhalation and external exposures.

There were no deaths attributable to radiation after the Fukushima accidents, either among workers or the public. In contrast, 134 of the workers at Chernobyl trying to quell the burning reactor developed acute radiation sickness (>2 Gy) and 28 died within a few months (Mettler et al., 2007). Many of these emergency workers and firefighters developed cataracts (UNSCEAR, 2011). Over 6000 cases of thyroid cancer have been observed among those exposed as children to radioactive iodines that were in contaminated milk that was not restricted, i.e., there was apparently little communication to tell the public not to drink milk. There was clear evidence of a dose response (Brenner et al., 2011) and the mean dose was very high at 650 mGy. In contrast the estimated thyroid dose from Fukushima exposures for 99% of the children measured closely after the accident was <4 mGy (Hosokawa et al., 2013).

MUCH IS KNOWN ABOUT RADIATION-INDUCED THYROID CANCER

Much is known about radiation-related thyroid cancer (Boice, 2005, 2006), from medical (Adams et al., 2010; Ron et al., 1989, 2012), Chernobyl (Brenner et al., 2011), and atomic bomb exposures (Furukawa et al., 2013). Radiation causes thyroid cancer, but not the next day and not within the next several years after exposure. There is a minimum latency, i.e., time from exposure to the development of detectable tumors, on the order of about 5 years. This is seen in practically all comprehensive, high-quality studies (Ron et al., 2012). Detecting radiation excesses within 1 or 2 years of exposure is not realistic, especially given the tiny-to-negligible doses received by practically all children. Thyroid cancer is caused by radiation, but not at tiny doses.

Radiation causes thyroid cancer, but primarily among those who are young at time of exposure, primarily under age 5 years and not among adults over age ~20 years (Ron et al., 2012). The screening survey found the opposite: no thyroid tumors were detected among children under the age of 5 years at the time of the NPP accident, and the detected tumors were all among the older children and teenagers who are at much lower risk (Suzuki et al., 2016; Wakeford, 2016).

RADIATION DOSE TO THE PUBLIC FROM THE FUKUSHIMA REACTOR ACCIDENT IS TINY

The World Health Organization (WHO, 2012, 2013), the United Nations Scientific Committee on the Effects of Atomic Radiation (UNSCEAR, 2013, 2014), the International Atomic Energy Agency (IAEA, 2014), and Fukushima Medical University (Ishikawa et al., 2015), measurements of children made shortly after the accident all point to extremely small population exposures (Hosokawa et al., 2013; Nagataki et al., 2013), and measurements of teenagers a few years later (Adachi et al., 2016) all point to extremely small population exposures. While estimates differ somewhat, from tiny to small, most are based on models and are much higher than the measured doses. Thus, care must be taken when evaluating the dose model (Nagataki and Takamura, 2016), and it would be my view to consider changing the models to become more in line with the measurements.

While there is a vanishingly small probability that any radiation-related cancers will result from the accident, environmental levels in some areas are not trivial and restrictions will be required for many years to come. While traveling to the NPP site after leaving J-Village (the sports complex-turned-staging-ground for workers hired to work on the crippled reactors), I noted monitors on the road started with 0.04 μSv h^{-1}. Normal background readings are about 0.01 μSv h^{-1}. Then the levels increased to 0.3 μSv h^{-1} and while there was traffic on the road there were no people in the towns we were passing. There were hardware stores, restaurants, and shopping centers, but they were uninhabited and grass and vines were growing everywhere. It was like the old movie *On the Beach* or the films on the rapture when everyone was taken and the towns were uninhabited. Then the level reached 0.5 μSv h^{-1}, then 0.7 μSv h^{-1}, and finally 0.9 μSv h^{-1} as we approached the plant. People are not allowed to return to their homes with such elevated background levels. In fact, 88,000 Japanese who were evacuated because of the NPP reactor accident may not be able to return for quite a long time.

SURVEYS ARE NOT SCIENTIFIC STUDIES

"After a nuclear accident, health surveys are very important and useful, but should not be interpreted as epidemiological studies. The results of such health surveys are intended to provide information to support medical assistance to the affected population" (IAEA, 2015).

There is little if any *scientific* reason to continue the screening activities, and certainly not for studying radiation effects. Doses are trivial and there is not enough statistical power to find an effect (even if there is one). All the surveys to date are noninformative with regard to a radiation association. However, there are public desires (e.g., mothers with young children), societal pressures, healthcare issues, and governmental responsibilities that will come into play in deciding whether to continue these surveys. If continued, it should be made very clear that this is a survey for the health of the people and not a scientific study. It would be to provide reassurance and for healthcare activities. Lumps and bumps would be detected by the ultrasensitive ultrasound devices, and tumors would be detected—caused by genetics or other factors, but not by radiation. Clear communication on the purpose of the screening survey and how to interpret outcomes is critical if they are to be continued. Studies are for science. Surveys are for people!

MENTAL HEALTH PROBLEMS ARE AN IMMEDIATE EFFECT FROM THE FUKUSHIMA ACCIDENT

Mental health problems are an important concern and have increased the rates of physical conditions as well. There is good evidence for raised rates of depression, anxiety, and medically unexplained physical symptoms in the populations in Fukushima Prefecture, especially among mothers of young children (Yoshida et al., 2016a; Goto et al., 2015; Boice, 2013) and even among public health nurses (Yoshida et al., 2016b). There is a concern over an increase in suicide rates (Ohto et al., 2015). The fear of radiation has no threshold as exemplified here where the estimated doses to children as well as mothers are tiny and could not be and will not be related to any future cancers— yet mental health problems are a serious consequence of the accident-related impact of this fear. It is important to remember that no radiation-related deaths or acute diseases have been observed among the workers and general public exposed to radiation from the Fukushima accident (UNSCEAR, 2013, 2014). Further, as summarized in UNSCEAR (2013), "The most important health effect is on mental and social well-being, related to the enormous impact of the earthquake, tsunami and nuclear accident, and the fear and stigma related to the perceived risk of exposure to ionizing radiation." Effects such as depression and posttraumatic stress symptoms have already been reported. The study by Yoshida and colleagues (2016a) on psychological stress continues to report severe mental problems. Thus, there is a need to continue to provide the Fukushima people with physical and mental support, as well as communicating effectively on the health risks of radiation. The lack of communication and the blur between a survey and a scientific study is increasing anxiety and the associated mental health problems. We need to improve the way we communicate. No one really cares how much you know unless they know how much you care. There is a need to be compassionate, to explain the radiation risks in a balanced way, and to engage at all times with the stakeholders (the local people in the various prefectures, hospitals, and medical care facilities), to be able to explain these important issues related to the health of the Fukushima people.

EXCESS THYROID CANCERS FROM SCREENING ARE AN ARTIFACT AND NOT RADIATION-RELATED

It is the general consensus that these detected tumors are related to the screening and not to radiation (Wakeford et al., 2016; Normile, 2016; Suzuki, 2016a,b; Nagataki and Takamura, 2016). Some of the tumors may never have come to clinical attention (overdiagnosis), and some may have come to clinical attention, but later (Vaccarella et al., 2016). When populations not within the Fukushima fallout areas were screened, thyroid tumor rates were comparable to those in the populations in the fallout areas, though numbers were small (Hayashida et al., 2015). The rates of detected thyroid tumors also did not vary by areas with different estimates of environment deposition, i.e., there was no ecological indication of a dose response (Ohira et al., 2016). The distribution of detected thyroid cancers were at ages greater than 5 years at exposure and concentrated among teenagers. Whereas for Chernobyl the distribution was concentrated among those under age 5 years (Suzuki et al., 2016; Wakeford, 2016;Takamura et al., 2016; Tronko et al., 2014). The age at exposure distribution from the screening survey is not consistent with the world's literature where the highest risk is among those <5 years at age of exposure, and very small among teenagers. Comprehensive screening studies in Korea have shown the effects of introducing thyroid screening programs into the population on a large scale. Substantial increases in thyroid cancer occurred among the entire population after the screening started, while the mortality rate stayed flat (Ahn et al., 2014). Similar results are reported in the United States (Davies and Welch, 2006). When population screening was reduced in Korea, the rates of thyroid cancer decreased (Ahn and Welch, 2015). Table 3.1 summarizes the evidence that the excess thyroid cancers detected from the screening survey is not due to radiation but to an overdiagnosis related to sensitive ultrasound screening examinations.

CONCLUSIONS

As summarized in Table 3.2, the following broad conclusions can be made.

Fukushima is not Chernobyl, neither in extent of radiation released nor health effects. Population doses from Fukushima are tiny and of little health consequence. The fear of radiation has caused immediate

Table 3.1 Why the thyroid results from the survey are not due to radiation and reflect "overdiagnosis" due to screening (see Vaccarella et al., 2016; Normile, 2016; Ahn et al., 2014, 2015)

- The thyroid risk is enormous—30–50 times normal population rates and is impossibly high
- Latency is too short and not consistent with the world's literature (<4 years is improbable to impossible)
- Age at exposure is not consistent with the world's literature where the highest risk is among those <5 years of age at exposure, and not among teenagers as reported in the screening survey
- Prevalence of thyroid cancer is the same regardless of regions within Fukushima Prefecture—no geographical variation by dose
- Similar screening results were found in areas not affected by radiation from Fukushima—screening not dose mattered
- Doses, measured, and modeled, are much too low to have any effect, now or in the future
- The IARC concludes that the screening excess of thyroid cancers is an artifact due to overdiagnosis from the very sensitive ultrasound technique used (Vaccarella et al., 2016)
- "A thyroid screening program would be expected to save lives by detecting cancers early, whether or not the cancers were caused by radioactivity" (Normile, 2016)
- In South Korea when screening was introduced in 2011, the rate of thyroid cancer diagnosis was 15 times what it was in 1993, yet there was no change in thyroid cancer mortality (Ahn et al., 2014)
- Similarly in the US, thyroid cancer incidence is increasing but with no change in mortality (Davies and Welch, 2006)
- Even though the vast majority of thyroid abnormalities are safe to ignore, "finding small lesions causes patients anxiety"
- The evidence suggests that thyroid growths among children are far more common than previously thought and must be considered normal. The Fukushima survey promises a "better understanding of the origins and development" of such growths and may lead to better treatment protocols
- Do not call the surveys studies; call them surveys. Studies are based on scientific methods, screening surveys are for the people

Table 3.2 Summary of Fukushima and thyroid cancer update

- Fukushima is not Chernobyl, neither in extent of radiation released nor health effects
- Population doses from Fukushima are tiny and of little health consequence
- The fear of radiation has caused immediate and lasting anxiety, affecting health
- When modeled doses differ from measured dose, change the model or use the measured values
- Do not misuse collective dose. It is wrong to multiply a trivial dose times a large population and compute theoretical numbers of cancers
- We know much about radiation-induced thyroid cancer from patients exposed for medical conditions, Chernobyl, and from atomic bomb survivors
  - Radiation causes thyroid cancer, but not immediately
  - Radiation causes thyroid cancer, but not after trivial doses, not detectable
  - Radiation causes thyroid cancer primarily among those <5 years at exposure and not among adults
- The screening survey does not indicate any radiation excess, but overdiagnosis due to the sensitive ultrasound screening
- Failure to communicate effectively contributed to the epidemic of thyroid cancer after Chernobyl, and the distrust of government after Fukushima and anxiety among the people
- Surveys are not for science but for the people
- Spend resources to address the serious mental health issues
- Engage with stakeholders at all times
- For future—Fund and train radiation professional education and provide job opportunities. In the US and other countries, the lack of trained radiation professionals indicates an existing crisis
- Be prepared now and when the next major nuclear incident comes along with effective and compassionate communication. No one cares how much you know, unless they know how much you care
- Be selective in the surveys you conduct and be clear in the goals, whether in the public interest to address societal concerns or in areas where new knowledge might be obtained such as stakeholder engagement, resettlement, mental health, remediation, mitigation, waste management, and more
- There remain many radiation protection and public health issues to address; choose wisely on how resources will be spent

and lasting anxiety affecting health. When modeled doses differ from measured dose, change the model. Do not misuse collective dose. It is wrong to multiply a trivial dose times a large population and compute theoretical numbers of cancers.

We know much about radiation-induced thyroid cancer from patients exposed for medical conditions, Chernobyl releases, and from atomic bomb survivors. Radiation causes thyroid cancer, but not immediately. Radiation causes thyroid cancer but not after trivial doses, and theoretical increases are not detectable. Radiation causes thyroid cancer primarily among those <5 years at exposure; and not among those over age ~ 20 years.

The screening survey does not indicate any radiation excess, but overdiagnosis due to ultrasound screening.

Failure to communicate effectively contributed to the epidemic of thyroid cancer after Chernobyl, and the distrust of the government after Fukushima and anxiety among the people.

In the USA and other countries, the lack of trained radiation professionals indicates an existing crisis. We need to train the young for the current and future needs in radiation science, and provide jobs!

Surveys are not for science but for people. Resources should be spent to address the serious mental health issues. Engage with stakeholders at all times. Be prepared now and when the next major nuclear incident comes along with better communications. No one cares how much you know, unless they know how much you care. Show compassion!

Do not call the surveys studies. Call them surveys. Be selective in the surveys you conduct and be clear in the goals. Whether in the public interest to address societal concerns or in areas where new knowledge might be obtained such as stakeholder engagement, resettlement, mental health, remediation, mitigation, waste management, and more. There remain many radiation protection and public health issues to address. Choose wisely. Thyroid and other cancers are not a health problem because, among other things, the doses to the public were tiny to nonexistent. The real problem is the anxiety, mental and associated physical health effects associated with the unbalanced fear of radiation (and perhaps the screening surveys per se when not clearly explained why they are conducted).

While the health effects possibly related to radiation exposure will be small to nonexistent, the economic burden, cleanup, and public anxiety may last for decades. The world needs to be aware of, concerned about, and helpful to the people of Fukushima.

REFERENCES

Adachi, N., Adamovitch, V., Adjovi, Y., Aida, K., Akamatsu, H., Akiyama, S., et al., 2016. Measurement and comparison of individual external doses of high-school students living in Japan, France, Poland and Belarus-the 'D-shuttle' project. J. Radiol. Prot. 36 (1), 49–66.

Adams, M.J., Shore, R.E., Dozier, A., Lipshultz, S.E., Schwartz, R.G., Constine, L.S., et al., 2010. Thyroid cancer risk 40 + years after irradiation for an enlarged thymus: an update of the Hempelmann cohort. Radiat. Res. 174 (6), 753–762.

Ahn, H.S., Kim, H.J., Welch, H.G., 2014. Korea's thyroid-cancer "epidemic"–screening and overdiagnosis. N. Engl. J. Med. 371 (19), 1765–1767.

Ahn, H.S., Welch, H.G., 2015. South Korea's thyroid-cancer "epidemic"--turning the tide. N. Engl. J. Med. 373 (24), 2389–2390.

Asia News Network (ANN), 2012. Disaster claimed 1,046 minors. March 8, 2012. [<http://news.asiaone.com/News/AsiaOne%2BNews/Asia/Story/A1Story20120308-332277.html> (accessed 16.01.17.)].

Boice Jr., J.D., 2005. Radiation-induced thyroid cancer – what's new? [Editorial]. J. Natl. Cancer Inst. 97, 703–704.

Boice Jr., J.D., 2006. Thyroid disease 60 years after Hiroshima and 20 years after Chernobyl. JAMA 295 (9), 1060–1062.

Boice Jr., J.D., 2012. Radiation epidemiology: a perspective on Fukushima. J. Radiol. Prot. 32, N33–N40.

Boice Jr., J.D., 2013. Fukushima conference in February 2013. Health Phys. News XLI (4), 13–15. [<http://ncrponline.org/wp-content/themes/ncrp/PDFs/BOICE-HPnews/11_Fukushima-Conf_Apr2013.pdf> (accessed 15.01.17.)].

Boice Jr., J.D., 2016. Fukushima--five years after: thyroid cancer. Health Phys. News XLIV (11), 20–21 [<http://ncrponline.org/wp-content/themes/ncrp/PDFs/BOICE-HPnews/52-Fukushima_Nov2016.pdf> (accessed 15.01.17.)].

Brenner, A.V., Tronko, M.D., Hatch, M., Bogdanova, T.I., Oliynik, V.A., Lubin, J.H., et al., 2011. I-131 dose response for incident thyroid cancers in Ukraine related to the Chornobyl accident. Environ. Health Perspect. 119 (7), 933–939.

Davies, L., Welch, H.G., 2006. Increasing incidence of thyroid cancer in the United States,1973-2002. JAMA 295 (18), 2164–2167.

Fukushima Medical University (FMU) and Nippon Foundation, 2015. 11–12 Sep 2011 1st International Expert Symposium in Fukushima. [<http://fmu-global.jp/workshop/symposium/11-12-sep-2011-1st-international-expert-symposium-in-fukushima/> (accessed 16.01.17.)].

Furukawa, K., Preston, D., Funamoto, S., Yonehara, S., Ito, M., Tokuoka, S., et al., 2013. Long-term trend of thyroid cancer risk among Japanese atomic-bomb survivors: 60 years after exposure. Int. J. Cancer 132, 1222–1226.

González, A.J., Akashi, M., Boice Jr., J.D., Chino, M., Homma, T., Ishigure, N., et al., 2013. Radiological protection issues arising during and after the Fukushima nuclear reactor accident. J. Radiol. Prot. 33 (3), 497–571.

Goto, A., Bromet, E.J., Fujimori, K., Pregnancy and Birth Survey Group of Fukushima Health Management Survey, 2015. Immediate effects of the Fukushima nuclear power plant disaster on depressive symptoms among mothers with infants: a prefectural-wide cross-sectional study from the Fukushima Health Management Survey. BMC Psychiatry 15, 59.

Hayashida, N., Imaizumi, M., Shimura, H., Furuya, F., Okubo, N., Asari, Y., et al., 2015. Thyroid ultrasound findings in a follow-up survey of children from three Japanese prefectures: Aomori, Yamanashi, and Nagasaki. Sci. Rep. 5, 9046.

Hosokawa, Y., Hosoda, M., Nakata, A., Kon, M., Urushizaka, M.A., Yoshida, M.A., 2013. Thyroid screening survey on children after the Fukushima Daiichi Nuclear Power Plant accident. Radiat. Emerg. Med. 2 (1), 82−86.

International Atomic Energy Agency (IAEA), 2014. The Follow-up IAEA International Mission on Remediation of Large Contaminated Areas Off-Site of the Fukushima Daiichi Nuclear Power Plant. NE/NEFW/2013. [<https://www.iaea.org/sites/default/files/final_report230114.pdf> (accessed 15.01.17.)].

IAEA), 2015. The Fukushima Daiichi accident. Report by the director general. Austria, IAEA. [<http://www-pub.iaea.org/MTCD/Publications/PDF/Pub1710-ReportByTheDG-Web.pdf> (accessed 15.01.17.)].

Ishikawa, T., Yasumura, S., Ozasa, K., Kobashi, G., Yasuda, H., Miyazaki, M., et al., 2015. The Fukushima Health Management Survey: estimation of external doses to residents in Fukushima Prefecture. Sci. Rep. 5, 12712.

Kamiya, K., Ishikawa, T., Yasumura, S., Sakai, A., Ohira, T., Takahashi, H., et al., 2016. External and internal exposure to Fukushima residents. Radiat. Prot. Dosim. 171 (1), 7−13.

Mettler Jr., F.A., Gus'kova, A.K., Gusev, I., 2007. Health effects in those with acute radiation sickness from the Chernobyl accident. Health Phys. 93 (5), 462−469.

Nagataki, S., Takamura, N., 2016. Radioactive doses - predicted and actual—and likely health effects. Clin. Oncol. (R. Coll. Radiol.) 28 (4), 245−254.

Nagataki, S., Takamura, N., Kamiya, K., Akashi, M., 2013. Measurements of individual radiation doses in residents living around the Fukushima Nuclear Power Plant. Radiat. Res. 180, 439−447.

Nippon Foundation, 2016. 5th International Expert Symposium in Fukushima on Radiation and HealthChernobyl + 30, Fukushima + 5 − Lessons and Solutions for Fukushima's Thyroid Question. [<http://www2.convention.co.jp/fukushima2016/english/index.html> (accessed 16.01.17.)].

Normile, D., 2016. Epidemic of fear. Science 351 (6277), 1022−1023.

Ohira, T., Takahashi, H., Yasumura, S., Ohtsuru, A., Midorikawa, S., Suzuki, S., et al., 2016. Comparison of childhood thyroid cancer prevalence among 3 areas based on external radiation dose after the Fukushima Daiichi nuclear power plant accident: The Fukushima health management survey. Medicine 95 (35), e4472.

Ohto, H., Maeda, M., Yabe, H., Yasumura, S., Bromet, E.E., 2015. Suicide rates in the aftermath of the 2011 earthquake in Japan. Lancet 385 (9979), 1727.

Ron, E., Modan, B., Preston, D., Alfandary, E., Stovall, M., Boice Jr., J.D., 1989. Thyroid neoplasia following low-dose radiation in childhood. Radiat. Res. 120 (3), 516−531.

Ron, E., Lubin, J.H., Shore, R.E., Mabuchi, K., Modan, B., Pottern, L.M., et al., 2012. Thyroid cancer after exposure to external radiation: a pooled analysis of seven studies. 1995. Radiat. Res. 178, AV43−AV60.

Suzuki, S., 2016a. Childhood and adolescent thyroid cancer in Fukushima after the Fukushima Daiichi Nuclear Power Plant Accident: 5 years on. Clin. Oncol. (R. Coll. Radiol.) 28 (4), 263−271.

Suzuki, S., 2016b. Re: Thyroid Cancer Among Young People in Fukushima. Epidemiology 27 (3), e19.

Suzuki, S., Suzuki, S., Fukushima, T., Midorikawa, S., Shimura, H., Matsuzuka, T., et al., 2016. Comprehensive survey results of childhood thyroid ultrasound examinations in Fukushima in the first four years after the Fukushima Daiichi Nuclear Power Plant accident. Thyroid 26 (6), 843−851.

Takamura, N., Orita, M., Saenko, V., Yamashita, S., Nagataki, S., Demidchik, Y., 2016. Radiation and risk of thyroid cancer: Fukushima and Chernobyl. Lancet Diabetes Endocrinol. 4 (8), 647.

Tokonami, S., Hosoda, M., Akiba, S., Sorimachi, A., Kashiwakura, I., Balonov, M., 2012. Thyroid doses for evacuees from the Fukushima nuclear accident. Sci. Rep. 2, 507.

Tronko, M.D., Saenko, V.A., Shpak, V.M., Bogdanova, T.I., Suzuki, S., Yamashita, S., 2014. Age distribution of childhood thyroid cancer patients in Ukraine after Chernobyl and in Fukushima after the TEPCO-Fukushima Daiichi NPP accident. Thyroid 24 (10), 1547−1548.

United Nations Scientific Committee on the Effects of Atomic Radiation (UNSCEAR), 2011. Sources and Effects of Ionizing Radiation, UNSCEAR 2008 Report (Scientific Annex D, Health effects due to radiation from the Chernobyl accident, Vol II). United Nations, New York.

United Nations Scientific Committee on the Effects of Atomic Radiation (UNSCEAR), 2013. Report of the United Nations Scientific Committee on the Effects of Atomic Radiation. Official Records of the General Assembly, Sixtieth Session (27-31 May 2013), Supplement No. 46. New York, United Nations. [<http://www.unscear.org/docs/GAreports/A-68-46_e_V1385727.pdf> (accessed 15.01.17.)].

United Nations Scientific Committee on the Effects of Atomic Radiation (UNSCEAR), 2014. 2013 Report Annex A: Levels and effects of radiation exposure due to the nuclear accident after the 2011 great East-Japan earthquake and tsunami. United Nations, New York. [<http://www.unscear.org/docs/reports/2013/13-85418_Report_2013_Annex_A.pdf> (accessed 15.01.17)].

Vaccarella, S., Franceschi, S., Bray, F., Wild, C.P., Plummer, M., Dal Maso, L., 2016. Worldwide thyroid-cancer epidemic? The increasing impact of vverdiagnosis. N. Engl. J. Med. 375 (7), 614−617.

Wakeford, R., 2016. Chernobyl and Fukushima-where are we now?. J. Radiol. Prot. 36 (2), E1−E5.

Wakeford, R., Auvinen, A., Gent, R.N., Jacob, P., Kesminiene, A., Laurier, D., et al., 2016. Re: Thyroid Cancer Among Young People in Fukushima. Epidemiology 27 (3), e20−e21.

World Health Organization (WHO), 2012. Preliminary dose estimation from the nuclear accident after the 2011 Great East Japan earthquake and tsunami. [<http://apps.who.int/iris/bitstream/10665/44877/1/9789241503662_eng.pdf?ua = 1> (accessed 15.01.17.)].

World Health Organization (WHO), 2013. Health risk assessment from the nuclear accident after the 2011 Great East Japan earthquake and tsunami, based on a preliminary dose estimation. World Health Organization, Geneva. [<http://apps.who.int/iris/bitstream/10665/78218/1/9789241505130_eng.pdf?ua = 1> (accessed 15.01.17.)].

Yamashita, S., Takamura, N., Ohtsuru, A., Suzuki, S., 2016. Radiation exposure and thyroid cancer risk after the Fukushima Nuclear Power Plant Accident in comparison with the Chernobyl Accident. Radiat. Prot. Dosim. 171 (1), 41−46.

Yasumura, S., Hosoya, M., Yamashita, S., Kamiya, K., Abe, M., Akashi, M., et al., 2012. Study protocol for the Fukushima Health Management Survey. J. Epidemiol. 22 (5), 375−383.

Yoshida, K., Shinkawa, T., Urata, H., Nakashima, K., Orita, M., Yasui, K., et al., 2016a. Psychological distress of residents in Kawauchi village, Fukushima Prefecture after the accident at Fukushima Daiichi Nuclear Power Station: the Fukushima Health Management Survey. Peer. J 4, e2353.

Yoshida, K., Orita, M., Goto, A., Kumagai, A., Yasui, K., Ohtsuru, A., et al., 2016b. Radiation-related anxiety among public health nurses in the Fukushima Prefecture after the accident at the Fukushima Daiichi Nuclear Power Station: a cross-sectional study. BMJ Open 6 (10), e013564.

CHAPTER 4

Reassessing the Capability to Attribute Pediatric Thyroid Cancer to Radiation Exposure: The FHMS Experience

Abel J. González
Argentine Nuclear Regulatory Authority, Buenos Aires, Argentina

INTRODUCTION

A response to the aftermath of the accident at the Fukushima Dai'ichi Nuclear Power Plant (hereinafter referred to as "the accident") was the launching of the Fukushima Health Management Survey (FHMS). The FHMS was originally designed as a health survey, namely as a systematic collection of factual data pertaining to health and disease in the population of Fukushima Prefecture, rather than as an epidemiological study, namely a study that compares two groups of people who are alike except for a factor such as exposure to radiation.

The FHMS main objective was a general examination and investigation of the health situation of people in the Prefecture with the objective inter alia of monitoring the residents' health conditions. It was aimed at disease prevention, early detection, and early medical treatment, thereby maintaining and promoting the residents' future health (FP, 2011; Yasumura, 2014). The FHMS was not designed to assess the attribution of effects to radiation from the accident.

Because of its findings on pediatric thyroid cancer incidence, however, the FHMS would also eventually lead to the so-called "*Fukushima thyroid question,*" namely whether a high incidence of this malignancy found by the survey was attributable to radiation exposure from the accident or to the survey itself.

The purpose of this chapter is to elucidate the Fukushima thyroid question by reassessing the epistemological capability of attributing pediatric thyroid cancer to radiation exposure. It takes into consideration the

Thyroid Cancer and Nuclear Accidents. DOI: http://dx.doi.org/10.1016/B978-0-12-812768-1.00004-6

experience accumulated by the FHMS, and also the information on attribution of radiation effects and inference of radiation risk reported by the United Nations Scientific Committee on the Effects of Atomic Radiation (UNSCEAR), to the United Nations General Assembly (UNGA), as well as specific epistemological difficulties for the unequivocal attribution of thyroid cancers.

THE FUKUSHIMA THYROID QUESTION

The elements associated to the FHMS, which would eventually lead to the Fukushima's thyroid question, could be summarized as follows:

1. The FHMS examined, with thyroid ultrasound screening, around 300,000 children living in the Fukushima Prefecture. Around 2100 of those presented thyroid nodules and were further examined using an advanced and highly sensitive ultrasound instrument. These examinations, complemented with further analyses, revealed around 100 cases of papillary thyroid cancers—a type of cancer that has been linked to radiation exposure. Thus, the overall prevalence of childhood papillary thyroid cancer in the Fukushima accident was determined to be around 37 per 100,000 (Susuki, 2015). This incidence is higher than the spontaneous incidence of pediatric thyroid cancers presumed at the time.

2. The surprisingly high incidence of pediatric thyroid cancer in Fukushima was viewed by some as a confirmation of early suspicions that there would be an increase in the incidence on this malignancy. The suspicions were based on initial convincing reasoning, as follows:
   - At the time of the Chernobyl accident, there had been a large increase in the thyroid cancer rate among children who drank milk highly contaminated with radioiodine. Following the accident there was a substantial environmental presence of radioiodines. Should children have incurred a significant intake of radioiodines, they would be at higher risk than adults. The effects would be detectable and attributable because the spontaneous incidence of thyroid cancer in children was presumed to be low and the sensitivity of children's thyroid glands to radiation was known to be high.
   - The World Health Organization had early estimated that for thyroid cancer, the estimated lifetime risk in females exposed by the

accident as infants could be predicted to increase by up to around 70% over baseline rates (WHO, 2013).

- Soon after the FHMS preliminary results were revealed, it was reported (in a peer-reviewed journal) that the excess of thyroid cancer that had been detected was unlikely to be explained by a screening surge (Tsuda, 2015).

3. All these elements contributed to create the perception that the excess in the incidence of pediatric thyroid cancers in the Fukushima area, which were being reported by the FHMS, should be attributable to radiation exposure from the accident.

4. However, many scientists observed other fundamental elements contradicting that initial perception, including the following:

- The thyroid doses incurred by children appeared to be low. As demonstrated in the aftermath of the Chernobyl accident, the main potential pathway for thyroid doses in children should have been the intake of milk containing radioiodine. However, following the accident, the typical intake of radioiodine via cow's milk was low owing to a number of factors including the following:

  - Dairy practices in Japan, such as generally sheltering cattle, prevented the ingestion of radioiodine by dairy cows;
  - The intake of radioiodine via milk was also limited by the relatively low contribution of milk to the diet of infants and by the strict restrictions on the consumption of milk imposed by the authorities following the accident; and,
  - While there were alternative iodine ingestion pathways, such as the consumption of leafy vegetables and drinking water, especially in the very early period following the release, the prompt restrictions on drinking water and food limited the intake via these pathways.

- As a result of these factors, the intake of radioiodine by children is likely to have been low (mainly attributable to inhalation) and, while there were uncertainties associated with the estimates in the first few days following the accident, the reported thyroid doses of children were unsurprisingly low.

- Thyroid cancer often causes no symptoms, thus going undiagnosed, and therefore the FHMS detections could well be due to the screening itself. In fact, similar results were obtained when the same screening was carried out on children living far away from the areas affected by the accident (Hayashida et al., 2015), and the proportion of suspicious or malignant cases was almost the same among regions in Fukushima Prefecture (FP, 2015).

- Previous experience has shown that the latency time for radiation induced thyroid cancer was longer than the 4 years that had elapsed since the accident, at the time of the FHMS reporting.
- The thyroid cancers found were in children in their late teenage years, but no cases were found in the most vulnerable group of infants. It is to be noted that the rates in this group were significantly elevated in the aftermath of the Chernobyl accident.

5. Following proper consideration of these elements and after detecting significant errors on the peer-reviewed assessments that attributed the FHMS increase to radiation from the accident, most scientists concluded that the incidence in Fukushima has turned out to be high simply due to the widespread screening (IAEA, 2015); namely, they considered that the FHMS may have ended up finding asymptomatic cancers that would have never been diagnosed should the FHMS not have been launched.

In sum, the main question that has been triggered by the FHMS can therefore be summarized in the following dilemma: Are the thyroid abnormalities being detected by the FHMS attributable to the radiation exposure caused by the Fukushima accident? Or are they revealing an important outcome of the FHMS, namely that the spontaneous incidence of thyroid abnormalities is larger than that previously presumed?

In order to address this important query it is necessary to revisit the epistemological limitations on the capability to attribute pediatric thyroid cancer to radiation exposure through health surveys and even in the course of proper epidemiological studies. Attribution requires demonstration and subsequent professional attestation that increases in incidence of this malignancy are due to radiation exposure. Thus, it is convenient to recall the main international judgment on the ability to attribute cancer to radiation exposure, which has been recently informed by UNSCEAR to UNGA (UNSCEAR, 2012). Since the capability to attribute pediatric thyroid cancers depends inter alia on the spontaneous incidence and radiosensitivity of this malignancy, it is also necessary to re-examine the apparently large variability and increasing tendency on the spontaneous incidence of the disease observed in populations in the absence of radiation exposure, and revisit relevant information on the radiation-related incidence (or radiosensitivity) of the disease.

UNSCEAR JUDGMENT ON ATTRIBUTABILITY

The 2012 UNSCEAR report to UNGA states inter alia that "increases in the incidence of health effects in populations cannot be attributed reliably to chronic exposure to radiation at levels that are typical of the global average background levels of radiation." The estimated thyroid doses incurred by children due to exposure to radioiodine in the aftermath of Fukushima were estimated to be relatively low, a tiny fraction of those incurred in Chernobyl (IAEA, 2015), and certainly the related effective doses were similar to background effective doses, therefore making attribution unfeasible. However, it can be argued that they were not "chronic," as radioiodines decay quickly, and that they are not comparable to background because background thyroid exposure to background radioiodine is basically nil.

However, in relation to the attribution of effects to individuals, UNSCEAR also warns that radiation-inducible malignancies suffered by individuals "cannot be unequivocally attributed to radiation exposure," regardless of the dose, "because radiation exposure is not the only possible cause and there are at present no generally available biomarkers that are specific to radiation exposure." It should be underlined that there are no known biomarkers able to identify that a given cancer has been cause by radiation exposure.

UNSCEAR also indicates nonetheless that "only if the spontaneous incidence of a particular type of stochastic effect were low and the radiosensitivity for an effect of that type were high (as is the case with some thyroid cancers in children) would the attribution of an effect in a particular individual to radiation exposure be plausible (or even ostensible), particularly if that exposure were high." But even then, UNSCEAR repeatedly warns, "the effect in an individual cannot be attributed unequivocally to radiation exposure, owing to competing possible causes."

In relation to collective attribution, namely the attribution of increases in the incidence of effects in an specifically studied cohort (such as that studied by the FHMS), UNSCEAR indicates that "an increased incidence of stochastic effects in a population could be attributed to radiation exposure through epidemiological analysis" (rather than through a survey)—"provided that, inter alia, the increased incidence of cases of the stochastic effect were sufficient to overcome the inherent statistical uncertainties." Only in this case, UNSCEAR cautions, "an increase in the incidence of stochastic effects in the exposed population could be properly verified and attributed to exposure." Again, for these cases of collective attribution, UNSCEAR notes that "if the spontaneous incidence of the effect in a population were low and the radiosensitivity for the relevant stochastic effect were high, an increase in the incidence of stochastic effects could at least be related to radiation, even when the number of cases was small."

In sum, UNSCEAR clearly indicates that individual attribution of cancers to radiation is unfeasible and the feasibility of collective attribution of cancers to radiation is intrinsically associated to the size of the cohort being studied, the level of dose incurred, and the radiosensitivity and the spontaneous incidence of the effect.

In fact, should the prevalent linear radiation-protection model on dose–response be assumed, attribution could typically be collectively proved if the number of subjects in the epidemiological cohort is higher than a number linked to the inverse of the square of the dose incurred through a parameter that is proportional to the spontaneous incidence and inversely proportional to the radiosensitivity (González, 2011, 2014a, b). While this approach can be disputed as a circular argument because it relies on a predetermined model of dose–response, UNSCEAR had implicitly used such a model in many of its estimates, although in its 2012 report it used a more basic statistical mathematics to express the lowest excess relative risk that could be seen for a given cohort, independent of dose and any presumed dose–response (UNSCEAR, 2012). It is nonetheless to be noted that, whatever approach is used for estimating the capability for attributing to radiation exposure the incidence of cancer in a cohort, in a given situation, such capability is directly related to the radiosensitivity and inversely related to the spontaneous incidence of the disease. In sum, the higher the radiosensitivity of the pediatric thyroid is, the easier it is to attribute to a radiogenic cause, but the greater the spontaneous incidence, the harder it is to attribute. i.e., if the incidence of thyroid cancer found by ultrasound is high, then the greater the chance of misattribution (in Fukushima) to radiation.

SPECIFIC DIFFICULTIES FOR ATTRIBUTING PEDIATRIC CANCERS TO RADIATION

Radiosensitivity

The radiosensitivity of pediatric thyroid cancer is very dependent on a number of factors, including age, sex, and local dietary circumstances and the estimates of the related risk are uncertain. These characteristics make attribution of this malignancy somehow cumbersome when the cohorts are not homogeneous.

Estimates on excess relative risk have been widely reported in the literature (e.g., Ron et al., 1995; Cardis et al., 2005; Ron, 2007). Nevertheless, such estimates include a significant factor of uncertainty: nominal risks have usually been estimated on the basis of epidemiological studies of populations exposed to high doses from external radiation rather than internal contamination and the relevant risk factor (which is used for radiation protection purposes) are mainly based on these studies (ICRP, 2005, 2007).

There are also estimations of risk based on internal exposure. Such information is mainly available from epidemiological studies performed in the aftermath of the Chernobyl accident and are summarized in this book (Chapter 1: Thirty Years After Chernobyl—Overview of the Risks of Thyroid Cancer, Based Upon the UNSCEAR Scientific Reports (2008–2012)). However these estimates involve dosimetric information with large uncertainties that are transmitted to the estimates of radiosensitivity.

Moreover, radiosensitivity depends very much on the availability in the diet of nonradioactive iodine, with a threefold increase in severely iodine-deficient areas (Holm, 2006).

In sum, while it is not a dominant factor in the limitations of attributability for pediatric thyroid cancers, uncertainties in the radiosensitivity of this malignancy certainly limit the capability of attribution.

Spontaneous Incidence

The main difficulty for attributing pediatric thyroid cancers is linked to the spontaneous incidence of this malignancy. In the aftermath of the Chernobyl accident, the locally reported spontaneous incidence of thyroid cancer in children was recorded to be very low (Williams et al., 1996). It is noted that, at the time, the methods used for detection were manual palpation rather than the ultrasound techniques now used, some of which were incorporated in the studies carried out in the aftermath of the accident. Many cancer cases were subsequently diagnosed and by 2008 UNSCEAR reported that a substantial increase in thyroid cancer incidence among persons exposed to the accident-related radiation as children or adolescents at the time of the accident had been observed in Belarus, Ukraine, and four of the more affected regions of the Russian Federation, indicating that, for the period 1991–2005, more than 6000 cases had been reported. While only 15 cases had proved fatal up to 2005, the thyroid cancer incidence continued to increase for this group (UNSCEAR, 2008). Given the presumed low spontaneous incidence of the malignancy, a substantial portion of these malignancies were collectively considered ostensibly attributable to radiation and de facto individually attributable also. In a very recent scientific gathering (Obninsk, 2016) new data were reported suggesting that the number of cases may be much higher. However, this finding is in a group of people now aged above 30 years old, where obviously the background incidence rate is much higher; it is therefore unclear which of these cases are attributable to radiation and which to spontaneous incidence.

A relatively new information on the spontaneous incidence of thyroid cancer is that, in most areas of the world, it is changing extensively, depending upon age and sex and, significantly, strongly on the quality and characteristic of the relevant screening. In fact, although mortality rates of thyroid cancers have kept nearly constant or been steadily declining, it appears that the spontaneous incidence has been increasing appreciably over the last few decades (Ferlay et al., 2014). While the declines in mortality might reflect changes in the diagnosis and treatment of the disease, the rise in incidence does not appear to reflect a real increase in the occurrence but is more likely due to a substantial increment in the detection of subclinical thyroid cancers through intensive screening over recent decades (La Vecchia et al., 2015). This is exactly what appears to have happened in the FHMS!

A typical example of this apparent surge has been recently reported (Ahn, 2014; Brito et al., 2016). Following a 1999 South Korean health program offering ultrasound thyroid screening, the rate of thyroid cancer diagnosis presented a 15-fold increase over 18 years, yet there was no change in thyroid cancer mortality. Eventually, it was shown that this apparent "epidemic" of thyroid cancer was due to screening (see Chapter 17: Thyroid Cancer Screening and Overdiagnosis in Korea).

The new available data on the spontaneous incidence and, in particular, the information arising from the FHMS may serve as a basis for revisiting the Chernobyl paradigm on ostensible attribution.

QUESTIONING THE PREDICTIONS ON ATTRIBUTION

The predictions on attribution to radiation of FHMS reported incidence of pediatric thyroid cancer have been questioned. The surge in incidence is being attributed to mass screening (Susuki, 2015). This seems to be substantiated not only by the UNSCEAR findings on attribution but also the thorough scientific examination of the FHMS data, comparisons with the outcome from Chernobyl studies, and the new international evidence on spontaneous incidence.

The scientific appropriateness of the peer-reviewed study that had implicitly attributed the increase to the Fukushima accident (Tsuda, 2015) was seriously challenged by many scientists (e.g., Jorgensen, 2016; Shibata, 2016; Takamura, 2016; Wakeford et al., 2016). They were swift and severe in criticizing a fundamental error in that the estimates compared the results of the FHMS results, which used advanced ultrasound devices that detect otherwise unnoticeable growths, with the few cases of thyroid cancer per million found by traditional clinical examinations of patients who have lumps or symptoms.

In its 2013 report UNSCEAR had concluded that, while there is a possibility that the risk of thyroid cancer among those children most exposed to radiation from the accident could increase, the occurrence of a large number of radiation-induced thyroid cancers in Fukushima Prefecture could be discounted (UNSCEAR, 2013). Moreover, UNSCEAR has recently confirmed that most new publications have reconfirmed the main assumptions and findings of its 2013 report, and none materially affected the main findings in, or challenged the major assumptions of, that report (UNSCEAR, 2016).

All in all, the large international study performed under the aegis of the International Atomic Energy Agency (IAEA), concluded that, conditional on the intense screening regime, the prevalence informed by the FHMS was considered "unlikely to be associated with radiation exposure from the accident and most probably denote the natural (i.e. spontaneous) occurrence of thyroid abnormalities in children." The study also concluded that "the abnormalities identified in the (FHMS) survey are unlikely to be associated with radiation exposure from the accident and most probably denote the natural occurrence of thyroid abnormalities in children of this age," and that, while uncertainties remained concerning the thyroid equivalent doses incurred by children immediately after the accident, "because the reported thyroid doses attributable to the accident were generally low, an increase in childhood thyroid cancer attributable to the accident is unlikely" (IAEA, 2015).

In sum, the thyroid abnormalities detected by the FHMS should not be associated with radiation exposure due to the accident. The incidence in Fukushima has turned out to be high simply due to the widespread screening, which may have ended up finding cancer that would have never caused a health problem for their entire lives even if left unattended.

THE CONSEQUENCES OF ERRONEOUS ATTRIBUTION

The incorrect attribution of the FHMS's reported cancers to the accident caused serious anguish among the parents of the affected children and has probably contributed to a major detrimental outcome from the accident, namely the psychological consequences observed in its aftermath.

In fact, UNSCEAR had concluded "the most important health effect [from the accident] is on mental and social well-being, related to (inter alia) the fear and stigma related to the perceived risk of exposure to ionizing radiation" (UNSCEAR, 2013). Coincidently, the group of experts convened by the IAEA to assess the radiological consequences from the accident had observed that the FHMS's Mental Health and Lifestyle Survey had shown associated psychological problems in some vulnerable groups of the affected population, such as increases in anxiety and posttraumatic stress disorders. Assessments of mental health status of children also suggested psychological difficulties (IAEA, 2015; Yabe et al., 2014).

At least one major lesson can be learned from the Fukushima thyroid question: international experts and organizations should be very careful and scientifically robust when attributing health effects to radiation exposure because wrong attribution might cause serious collateral damage. The time is ripe to reiterate the fact that false attribution of effects to radiation is linked to the so-called "*dead-body* factor" (González, 2007). This is the assignment of casualties to radiation exposure without scientific proof followed by proper professional attestation, which causes serious psychological consequences for those affected.

CONCLUSION: NEW LIGHTS ON ATTRIBUTION FROM THE FHMS FINDINGS

The Fukushima thyroid question is being resolved and new lights on attribution are being provided. The FHMS reported surge in the incidence of pediatric thyroid cancers is seemingly due to screening rather than to radiation exposure to the accident. Notwithstanding, the FHMS findings also elucidate on the higher than expected spontaneous incidence of pediatric thyroid cancers.

These findings should trigger research on the epidemiological ability to attribute unequivocally incidences of this malignancy to radiation by reassessing the epistemological limits of its epidemiological attribution. In the aftermath of a nuclear accident, the simplistic approach of considering most pediatric thyroid cancers to be de facto ostensibly attributable to radiation exposure ought to be revisited.

The time seems to be ripe for recalling an important conclusion of the membership of the Task Group convened by the International Commission on Radiological Protection for compiling lessons learned from the accident: "the radiological protection community has the responsibility, if not the ethical duty, to learn from the Fukushima accident and suggest improvements in the system of protection. Accordingly, it should be ensured that [inter alia] the limitations of epidemiological studies for attributing radiation effects... be clearly explained..." (González et al., 2013).

REFERENCES

Ahn, H.S., Kim, H.J., Welch, H.G., 2014. Korea's thyroid-cancer "epidemic"—screening and overdiagnosis. N. Engl. J. Med. 371, 1765–1767.

Brito, J.P., Kim, H.J., Han, S.J., Lee, Y.S., Ahn, H.S., et al., 2016. Geographic distribution and evolution of thyroid cancer epidemic in South Korea. Thyroid 26 (6), 864–865.

Cardis, E., Kesminiene, A., Ivanov, V., et al., 2005. Risk of thyroid cancer after exposure to 131I in childhood. J. Natl. Cancer Inst. 97, 724–732.

Ferlay, J., Bray, F., Steliarova-Foucher, E. (Eds.), 2014. Cancer Incidence in Five Continents, CI5plus: IARC Cancer Base No. 9 [Internet]. International Agency for Research on Cancer, Lyon, France.

Fukushima Prefecture, 2011. Terms of Reference of the Committee for the Fukushima Health Management Survey.

Fukushima Prefecture, Proc. 18th Prefectural Oversight Committee Meeting for Fukushima Health Management Survey, Fukushima, Japan, 12 February 2015.

González, A.J., 2007. Chernobyl vis-à-vis the nuclear future: an international perspective. Health Phys. 93 (5), 571–592.

González, A.J., 2011. Epistemology on the attribution of radiation risks and effects to low radiation dose exposure situations. Int. J. Low Radiat. 8 (3).

González, A.J., 2014a. Clarifying the paradigm on radiation effects & safety management: UNSCEAR report on attribution of effects and inference of risks. Nucl. Eng. Technol. 46 (4).

González, A.J., 2014b. Clarifying the paradigm for protection against low radiation doses: retrospective attribution of effects vis-á-vis prospective inference of risk. Radiat. Prot. Australas. 31 (2).

González, A.J., Akashi, M., Boice Jr., J.D., Chino, M., Homma, T., Ishigure, N., et al., 2013. Radiological protection issues arising during and after the Fukushima nuclear reactor accident. J. Radiol. Prot. 33 (3), 497–571.

Hayashida, N., Imaizumi, M., Shimura, H., Furuya, F., Okubo, N., Asari, Y., et al., 2015. Thyroid ultrasound findings in a follow-up survey of children from three Japanese Prefectures: Aomori, Yamanashi, and Nagasaki. Sci. Rep. 5, 9046. Available from: http://dx.doi.org/10.1038/srep09046.

Holm, L.E., 2006. Thyroid cancer after exposure to radioactive 131I. Acta Oncol. 45 (8), 1037–1040.

IAEA, 2015. International Atomic Energy Agency. The Fukushima Daiichi Accident (Non-serial Publication). Report by the Director General and five technical volumen. Subject Classification: 0610-Accident response STI/PUB/1710; ISBN:978-92-0-107015-9. IAEA.

International Commission on Radiological Protection. Low-Dose Extrapolation of Radiation-Related Cancer Risk. ICRP Publication 99, Ann. ICRP 35 4. (2005).

International Commission on Radiological Protection. The 2007 Recommendations of the International Commission on Radiological Protection. ICRP Publication 103, Ann. ICRP 37 2–4. (2007).

Jorgensen, T.J., 2016. Re: Thyroid cancer among young people in Fukushima. Epidemiology 27 (3), e17.

La Vecchia, C., Malvezzi, M., Bosetti, C., Garavello, W., Bertuccio, P., Levi, F., et al., 2015. Thyroid cancer mortality and incidence: a global overview. Int. J. Cancer 136, 2187–2195.

Obninsk, 2016. International Conference on Health Effects of Chernobyl: Prediction and Actual Data-30 Years after the Accident. Obninsk, Russia, May 17–19, 2016. http://radiation-and-risk.com/index.php/en/info-letter.

Ron, E., 2007. Thyroid cancer incidence among people living in areas contaminated by radiation from the Chernobyl accident. Health Phys. 93, 502–511.

Ron, E., Lubin, J.H., Shore, R.E., et al., 1995. Thyroid cancer after exposure to external radiation: a pooled analysis of seven studies. Radiat. Res. 141, 259–277.

Shibata, Y., 2016. Re: Thyroid cancer among young people in Fukushima. Epidemiology 27 (3), e19–e20.

Susuki, S., 2015. Childhood and adolescent thyroid cancer in Fukushima after the Fukushima Daiichi nuclear power plant accident: 5 Years on. Clin. Oncol. 28, 263–271.

Takamura, N., 2016. Re: Thyroid cancer among young people in Fukushima. Epidemiology 27 (3), e18.

Tsuda, et al., 2015. Thyroid cancer detection by ultrasound among residents ages 18 years and younger in Fukushima, Japan: 2011 to 2014. Epidemiology 27 (3), 316–322. Available from: http://dx.doi.org/10.1097/EDE.0000000000000385.

UNSCEAR, (2008). Report of the United Nations Scientific Committee on the Effects of Atomic Radiation Fifty-sixth session (Vienna, 10–18 July 2008) to the UN General Assembly. Official Records Sixty-third Session. Supplement No. 46. Document A/63/46.

UNSCEAR, (2012). *Report of the United Nations Scientific Committee on the Effects of Atomic Radiation Fifty-ninth session* (Vienna, 21–25 May 2012) to the UN General Assembly Sixty-seventh session. Official Records. Supplement No. 46. Document A/67/46.

UNSCEAR, (2013). Official records of the General Assembly, Sixty-eighth Session, Supplement No. 46 and corrigendum (A/68/46 and Corr.1); and, *Sources, Effects and Risks of Ionizing Radiation. Volume 1: Report to the General Assembly and Scientific Annex A: Levels and Effects of Radiation Exposure due to the Nuclear Accident after the 2011 Great East-Japan Earthquake and Tsunami.* UNSCEAR 2013 Report. United Nations Scientific Committee on the Effects of Atomic Radiation. United Nations sales publication. E.14.IX.1. United Nations, New York, 2014.

UNSCEAR, (2016). UNSCEAR. *Report of the United Nations Scientific Committee on the Effects of Atomic Radiation.* Sixty-third session (Vienna, 27 June–1 July 2016) to the Seventy-first session of the UN General Assembly Document A/71/46.

Wakeford, R., Auvinen, A., Gent, R.N., Jacob, P., Kesminiene, A., Laurier, D., et al., 2016. Re: Thyroid Cancer Among Young People in Fukushima. Epidemiology 27 (3), e20–e21.

Williams E.D. et al., 1996. Effects on the thyroid in populations exposed to radiation as a result of the chernobyl accident. In: Proceedings of the International Conference on One Decade After Chernobyl: Summing Up the Consequences of the Accident held in Vienna, Austria, 8–12 April 1996. IAEA Proceedings Series, ISSN 0074-1884. IAEA, Vienna, 1996, pp. 207–230.

World Health Organization, 2013. ISBN 978 92 4150513 0 (NLM classification: WN 665). Health Risk Assessment from the Nuclear Accident after the 2011 Great East Japan Earthquake and Tsunami, Based on a Preliminary Dose Estimation. World Health Organization, Geneva.

Yabe, H., Suzuki, Y., Mashiko, H., Nakayama, Y., Hisata, M., Niwa, S., et al., 2014. Psychological distress after the Great East Japan Earthquake and Fukushima Daiichi nuclear power plant accident: results of a Mental Health and Lifestyle Survey through the Fukushima Health Management Survey in FY2011 and FY2012, Fukushima. J. Med. Sci. 60 (1), 57–67.

Yasumura S., 2014. Overview of Fukushima Health Management Survey, The Third International Expert Symposium in Fukushima: Beyond Radiation and Health Risk—Toward Resilience and Recovery. Fukushima, Japan.

FURTHER READING

Sasakawa, Y., 2012. International Expert Symposium in Fukushima. J. Radiol. Prot. 32 (1), (see also Conclusions and Recommendations of the International Expert Symposium in Fukushima: Radiation and Health Risks, *J. Radiol. Prot.* **31** (4) (2011), 381).

Suzuki, S., Satoru, S., Toshihiko, F., Sanae, M., Hiroki, S., Takashi, M., et al., 2016. Thyroid 26 (6), 843–851.

Yamashita, S.I., Suzuki, S., et al., 2013. Risk of thyroid cancer after the Fukushima nuclear power plant accident. Respir. Investig. 51 (3), 128–133.

Yasumura, S., Hosoya, M., Yamashita, S., Kamiya, K., Abe, M., Akashi, M., et al., 2012. Study protocol for the Fukushima Health Management Survey. J. Epidemiol. 22 (5), 375–383.

PART II

Chernobyl + 30

Post-Chernobyl Pediatric Papillary Thyroid Carcinoma in Belarus: Histopathological Features, Treatment Strategy, and Long-Term Outcome

Yuri E. Demidchik[1,2], Mikhail V. Fridman[1,8], Svetlana Mankovskaya[1,3], Olga Krasko[3], Kurt W. Schmid[4], Alfred K. Lam[5], Pavel Moiseev[6], Vladimir A. Saenko[7] and Shunichi Yamashita[7]

[1]Republican Centre for Thyroid Tumors, Minsk, Belarus [2]Belarusian Medical Academy of Postgraduate Education, Minsk, Belarus [3]National Academy of Sciences of Belarus, Minsk, Belarus [4]University of Duisburg-Essen, Essen, Germany [5]Griffith University, Gold Coast, QLD, Australia [6]Republican Scientific Practical Centre of Oncology and Medical Radiology named after N.N. Aleksandrov, Minsk, Belarus [7]Nagasaki University, Nagasaki, Japan [8]Minsk Municipal Clinical Oncological Dispensary, Minsk, Belarus

Thirty years ago, an explosion and subsequent fire destroyed the reactor unit No. 4 at the Chernobyl Nuclear Power Station in northern Ukraine, which led to the release of a large amount of radioactive materials into the environment. The highest levels of contamination occurred in the southern regions of Belarus. A sharp increase in thyroid cancer incidence in Belarusian children and adolescents was an object of attention of the scientific and medical community during all this time. Before the Chernobyl accident, the experience in pediatric papillary thyroid carcinoma (PTC) was rather limited across the world. Therefore, the lessons learned in the course of comprehensive multidisciplinary investigations of the long-term effects of internal irradiation on children were in demand for medical practice. This review analyzes the major results of clinical and morphological studies, and recent trends that determine the direction of future investigations.

POST-CHERNOBYL PEDIATRIC THYROID CANCER

Epidemiology

Investigations into thyroid cancer related to the Chernobyl accident paid particular attention to children, as they are the most vulnerable

Thyroid Cancer and Nuclear Accidents. DOI: http://dx.doi.org/10.1016/B978-0-12-812768-1.00005-8

group with the highest risk of developing thyroid malignancy after exposure. The first signs of the increase in thyroid cancer incidence in children and adolescents exposed to Chernobyl fallout was observed in 1990–91. A strong dose relationship was found between radiation exposure and the risk of developing thyroid cancer, with an odds ratio (OR) of 5.5 at 1 Gy. Also, a strong link between young age at exposure and the risk of developing thyroid cancer was established (Kenigsberg et al., 2002).

According to the Belarusian Cancer Registry, in the second half of the first decade after the Chernobyl accident (1990–95), the incidence of PTC reached 59.52 and 61.09 per 100,000 in prepubertal children (aged ≤ 10 years old), and in older (peripubertal) children (11–14 years old), respectively; most cases were from the southern areas of Belarus. From 1996 to 2001, the incidence rates were 58.78 and 69.66 per 100,000 in 11–14- and 15–18-year-old age groups, respectively. Finally, during the period 2002–05 only adolescent cases were diagnosed with the incidence of 45.56 per 100,000 individuals.

According to the Childhood Cancer Sub-Registry of Belarus, where all information on children diagnosed/treated for any type of tumor in the country is entered, 1078 children <19 years old with all types of PTC born before April 1, 1987, were registered in Belarus during the period of "radiogenic thyroid cancer" from January 1, 1990 to March 31, 2005. Patients with radiation history were identified according to medical, demographic, and geographical data. All our patients who were children (<14 years old) by April 26, 1986, were exposed to radiation after the accident under various circumstances and to various amounts of ^{131}I.

Initial Treatment

All patients in the study underwent surgery according to the known extent of disease at the time of diagnosis. In the early 1990s, surgeons preferred thyroid lobectomy or subtotal thyroidectomy. Neck lymph node dissection was performed when enlarged lymph nodes were present. Lymph node dissection also was done based on operative findings suggestive of their involvement. All patients who were treated with lateral lymph node resection also had central neck dissection. Since 1998, total thyroidectomy (TT) has been the standard operation (Demidchik et al., 2006) in line with the national guidelines, in either a one- or two-step procedure (the latter was performed when fine-needle aspiration findings were indeterminate and PTC was diagnosed on pathology), with bilateral (levels II–IV) and central (level VI) cervical lymph node dissection. In addition, postoperative ^{131}I ablation of thyroid remnants or distant metastases was performed 4–6 weeks after surgery, followed by hormone suppression therapy with a mean dose of 2.5 μg of levothyroxine per kg of body weight (Demidchik et al., 2006).

In Belarus, our approach to management of PTC in children and adolescents was the following.

1. TT is the only initial surgical approach. A small unilateral tumor in the thyroid should not be treated alternatively because the preoperative evaluation cannot discriminate between PTC confined to the gland and a neoplasm with minimal extrathyroidal extension.
2. If a compartment-oriented central and ipsilateral lymph node dissection was not performed during the initial surgery, risk of nodal disease based on age and morphological specifications should be evaluated to make a decision regarding the repeated surgery. For example, in our experience, central and bilateral cervical lymph nodes are frequently involved in cases of diffuse sclerosing variant of PTC or when the tumor localizes in close proximity to the isthmus and is accompanied by intrathyroidal lymphogenic psammoma bodies.
3. Treatment of childhood PTC needs special expertise not only from a skillful thyroid surgeon but also from an experienced thyroid pathologist specialized in this very specific area.
4. Vascular invasion, young age at diagnosis, and radioactive iodine therapy not performed during the initial management increase the risk of distant recurrence in children after TT. Therefore, children and adolescents with PTC could be assigned to two risk groups: those in whom all three risk factors are absent (low risk) and those in whom at least one factor presents (high risk).

Clinical and Morphological Features

Histological slides were available for 936 patients with PTC, who were included in the analysis of clinical and pathological data (Figs. 5.1 and 5.2).

Three age subgroups were considered: ≤ 10 years old or young children, $n = 157$ (16.8%), 11–14 years old or peripubertal children, $n = 364$ (38.9%), and 15–18 years old or adolescents, $n = 415$ (44.3%).

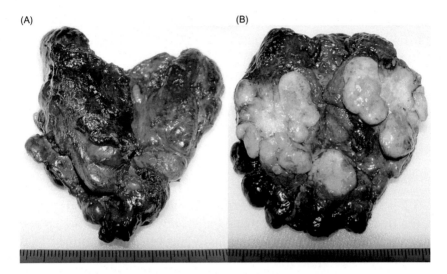

Figure 5.1 Childhood macrometastatic PTC with extranodal extension, gross pathology. (A) A bulky tumor almost completely occupying the thyroid lobe; enlarged central cervical lymph nodes bound to local tissues. (B) A gray-white solid multilobular lesion in the thyroid lobe (same case, sagittal view).

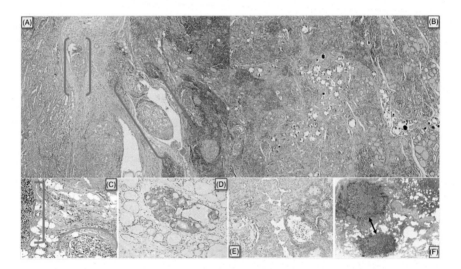

Figure 5.2 Characteristic microscopic features of childhood PTC. (A) Solid architectonic (may be observed as a tumor area or be the dominant pattern), infiltrative growth, and intraglandular blood vessel invasion (×40, small veins with tumor emboli marked with green brackets). (B) Numerous psammoma bodies permeating lymphatic vessels (×40). (C) Extrathyroidal extension to the fat tissue (×100, tumor complex [encircled] located in the proximity of the parathyroid gland [marked with a green bracket]). (D) Intrathyroidal spread with small tumor foci in the connective tissue septa (×200, tumor cells stained with CK19 antibody). (E) Lymph node metastasis in a patient with diffuse sclerosing variant of PTC featuring classical thyroglobulin-positive papillary structures coexisting with thyroglobulin-negative squamous cells metaplastic foci (×200). (F) Miliary pulmonary metastases (double arrow) frequently seen in childhood PTCs (×40). Hematoxylin and eosin staining (A, B, C, F); immunohistochemistry for CK19 (D) and thyroglobulin (E).

Female patients were more prevalent in all age subgroups (male/female ratios 1:1.6, 1:1.6, and 1:2.0, respectively). Patients in the youngest age group, as compared with older children and adolescents, had regional (N1) and distant (M1) metastases ($P < 0.001$) more frequently. Classical and solid variants of PTC ($P < 0.001$), nonencapsulated tumors ($P < 0.001$), and solid and follicular growth pattern ($P < 0.001$) were also more frequent in young children. In addition, PTC in the youngest patients featured extensive intratumoral fibrosis ($P = 0.006$), blood vessel invasion ($P = 0.014$), peritumoral/intraglandular psammoma bodies ($P = 0.002$), and lymphatic invasion ($P < 0.001$). Intrathyroidal spread ($P < 0.001$), multifocal growth ($P = 0.037$), and coexisting thyroid diseases ($P < 0.001$) were typical for adolescents. Most tumors displayed extrathyroidal extension corresponding to pT3–T4 category: 57/157 (36.3%) in the young children group, 164/364 (45.0%) in peripubertal children and 166/415 (40.0%) in adolescents. Interestingly, tumor size in patients with post-Chernobyl PTC was rather small: mean 14.4 mm, and not exceeding 10 mm in 41.2% of patients. Regional lymph nodes were involved in 691 (73.7%), and distant metastases were detected in 104 (11.1%) of patients (Fridman et al., 2014).

In order to identify parameters significantly associated with local, regional, and advanced disease, both bivariate and multivariate analyses were performed. The strongest factor for extrathyroidal extension was the absence of tumor capsule (infiltrative growth) or diffuse intrathyroidal spread (OR = 9.48, 95%CI = 3.50–30.73), for nodal disease—lymphatic vessel invasion (OR = 23.41, 95%CI = 11.66–50.84), and for distant metastases—lateral lymph node involvement (OR = 6.08, 95% CI = 3.43–11.31) (Fridman et al., 2014).

The comparative analysis of clinical and morphological features of PTC in irradiated children and teenagers was carried out with regard to the duration of the latent period. Patients operated during the (first) period from January 1990 to December 1995 had a comparatively low frequency of lateral nodal disease (34.6% vs. 37.5% and 49.0% for patients operated in 1996–1999 and 1999–2005, respectively). Also, a lower rate of lymph node metastases (N1a + N1b) was found in patients with papillary microcarcinomas (50.8% vs. 59.8% and 60.5%). On the other hand, a tendency for distant metastases was revealed. In children and adolescents operated during the (second) period from January 1996 to May 1999, there was a disproportionately low frequency of lateral lymph node metastases (37.5%) and a higher rate of distant metastases (13.5%). There were varying frequencies of N1b and M1 during two other periods: 34.6% and 14.4% in 1990–1995, and 49.0 and 5.4% during 1999–2005. Interestingly, there was no difference in clinical presentation of patients with PTC in the post-Chernobyl subgroup operated during the last (third) period from June 1999 to September 2005, as compared to their counterparts from the sporadic group matched by age and gender (Fridman et al., 2015a).

Genetic Data

RET protooncogene is known to play an important role in the pathogenesis of PTC. Several groups have investigated the relationship between morphological subtypes of PTC and molecular pathology. All have found that the solid type of PTC is associated with the presence of *RET/PTC3*, and the classic type with *RET/PTC1* (Nikiforov, 2002; Thomas et al., 1999). Our own pilot study of 17 patients (9 girls and 8 boys; age 14.0–17.3 years old) with post-Chernobyl tumors and 35 patients (22 girls and 13 boys; age 7.0–18.0 years old) with sporadic tumors showed that *RET/PTC* rearrangements were detected overall in 18 of 52 samples (34.6%) (unpublished data). In post-Chernobyl cases, *RET/PTC* rearrangements were identified in seven of 17 (41.2%) patients, including *RET/PTC1*—4 (23.5%), and *RET/PTC3*—3 (17.6%). These fusions were revealed in 11 of 35 cases (31.4%) of sporadic pediatric PTC: *RET/PTC1* in seven (20.0%) and *RET/PTC3* in four (11.4%) tumors. The results show no significant difference in the prevalence of *RET/PTC* between different etiological forms of PTC in young patients. However, definitive conclusions could not be drawn because of the relatively small sample size. Of note, *RET/PTC* rearrangements were associated with larger tumors ($P = 0.0138$), nodal disease (100.0% vs. 73.5%, $P = 0.0195$), and distant metastases to the lung ($P = 0.0152$). *RET/PTC*-positive tumors displayed an aggressive biological behavior: extrathyroidal extension (13 of 18, 72.2%), lymphatic vessel invasion (18 of 18, 100%), psammoma bodies (17 of 18, 94.4%) that corresponded well to the high rate of lymph node (100%) and distant (27.8%) metastases.

Also, a comparative analysis showed the differences in tumor growth pattern between the groups. Classic or diffuse sclerosing PTC was frequently *RET/PTC1*-positive. Solid or follicular architectonics correlated with *RET/PTC3* positivity.

Follow-Up

The 20-year treatment results were evaluated for 1078 post-Chernobyl patients using hospital records and cancer registry. The outcomes during the study period were as follows: 974 (90.4%) of patients had complete clinical remission and 77 (7.1%) had relapses (loco-regional—42, distant—35). Since 1990, 21 patients (1.9%) died: one from advanced disease, one from pulmonary fibrosis after multiple radioiodine therapy courses (17 GBq in total) and intrapleural chemotherapy, three from secondary malignancies, and three from other internal diseases such as cardiac failure, liver cirrhosis, and myxedema due to an inadequate levothyroxine intake after TT; seven committed suicide, and six died due to accidents/traumas. Overall survival was 96.9% with a median follow-up of 16.21 (range 7.8–23.1) years. The 20-year event-free survival and relapse-free survival were 87.8% and 92.3%, respectively, with a median follow-up of 15.36 years (Fridman et al., 2014).

Thus, the outcome of PTC both in children and in adolescents exposed to the post-Chernobyl radioiodine fallout was rather favorable: TT with radioiodine treatment is recommended for minimizing locoregional or distant recurrence. Disease-free survival after TT at 5, 10, and 20 years was 97.8% ± 0.6%, 97.0% ± 0.7%, and 97.0% ± 0.7%, respectively. For comparison, disease-free survival after non-TT at 5, 10, and 20 years was 92.8% ± 1.5%, 88.3% ± 1.9%, and 84.5% ± 2.2%, respectively. However, even after TT, the chance of recurrence exists, and tumor may relapse within ∼5 years. If TT was not performed, the probability of recurrence is higher and persists for ∼20 years (Fridman et al., 2014).

Currently, there is no technique to identify unambiguously extrathyroidal extension and/or lymph node metastasis except for cases with overt signs; therefore, these risk factors for recurrence cannot be detected/ruled out prior to surgery. Therefore, we propose to assign all patients aged ≤18 years to the moderate-risk group and those who were diagnosed with lateral nodal disease and distant metastasis in the high-risk group.

Our results support previously published observations that PTC developed after internal exposure to radioiodine does not display specific risk factors for recurrence that are different from those in sporadic PTC. Consequently, common treatment approaches for patients with

PTC should be recommended, regardless of history of radiation exposure (Rumyantsev et al., 2011).

The proponents for TT usually advocate this approach because it enables correct tumor staging as well as conditions patient for radioiodine treatment. The clinical situation in children is more complicated: we should consider that children and adolescents with PTC have a substantial risk for extrathyroidal extension. For example, in a reference cohort of patients with sporadic PTC, 45.5% had extrathyroidal extension and/or lymph node metastasis, and 27.3% of tumors were sized ≤ 10 mm. In our study, nodal disease was found in 71.6% of patients with sporadic PTC, and 62.5% of tumors sized ≤ 10 mm (Fridman et al., 2016).

During the up to 15 years-long follow-up, the prevalence of second primary malignancies (SPM) in young adults treated for post-Chernobyl PTC is 1%. Additional malignancies were more prevalent in female patients: 28/41 (68.3%). Cervical ($n = 7$), breast ($n = 4$), and colon ($n = 4$) cancers were the most common solid tumors. In 18 out of 41 (43.9%) cases, SPM was diagnosed in the same year as PTC. Metachronous malignancies were mostly revealed during the first decade of observation (18/23), among which cervical cancer ($n = 4$) and melanoma ($n = 3$) were most frequent. Thus, post-Chernobyl PTC survivors are at risk of developing SPM of different tissues; nine patients (22.0%) died of it (Fridman et al., 2015b).

Recent Data

Our current research is focusing on the young adult patients who were exposed to post-Chernobyl radiation during childhood and treated in Belarus for PTC during the years 2003–2013. The study subjects ($n = 359$, 81 males and 278 females, male/female ratio 1/3.4) were born between January 1, 1984 and March 31, 1987 (i.e., aged 0–2 years at the time of the Chernobyl accident) and were ≥ 19 years old at surgery. The details of patients' presentations, radiation history, surgical and pathological findings, and survival outcome were obtained from medical records (Fridman et al., 2016).

From the epidemiological point of view, a clear increase in thyroid cancer incidence is seen in the post-Chernobyl young adult population. For patients born between January 1, 1984 and March 31, 1987, the crude incidence rate group ranged from 25 cases per million for individuals aged 20–24 years to 26 cases per million in those aged 25–29 years. According to the Belarusian Cancer Registry, such a rate is 2.5 times higher than that in the 19–24-year-old age group of subjects born during the period from January 1, 1988 to March 31, 1990 (i.e., not exposed to Chernobyl fallouts), which is 10.3 per million.

Several morphological and clinical characteristics were found to associate with different histological variants of PTC. In conventional and oncocytic variants, the prevalence of extrathyroidal extension, nodal disease, nonencapsulated tumors, and lymphatic vessel invasion was above 50%, and it was even higher in tall cell or diffuse sclerosing variants. It is noteworthy that nearly all patients with distant metastases had the diffuse sclerosing variant of PTC; in our opinion, it is highly possible that in this variant the tumor disseminates to the lungs via lymphatic vessels. Extrathyroidal extension was strongly associated with lymph node ($P < 0.001$) and distant ($P = 0.015$) metastases, diffuse sclerosing and tall cell variants ($P < 0.001$) and occurrence of solid architecture, subcapsular localization, and extensive intratumoral fibrosis ($P < 0.001$), vascular invasion and the presence of psammoma bodies ($P < 0.001$), extensive mononuclear infiltration and a low frequency of background pathology ($P < 0.001$). On the other hand, small-size tumors confined to the thyroid (pT1a), were usually localized inside the thyroid lobe (64.7%), had conventional histological pattern (the admixture of the papillary and follicular architectonic) (82.4%), and had follicular adenoma (6.5%) or goiter (22.5%) as concomitant thyroid diseases. Nevertheless, small tumors frequently metastasized to the regional lymph nodes (35.3% and 37% for pT1a and pT1b/pT2 stages, respectively) (Fridman et al., 2016).

CONCLUSION

The phenomenon of post-Chernobyl thyroid cancer continues to exist and needs further investigation to better clarify the consequences of the Chernobyl accident for human health.

REFERENCES

Demidchik, Y.E., Demidchik, E.P., Reiners, C., Biko, J., Mine, M., Saenko, V.A., et al., 2006. Comprehensive clinical assessment of 740 cases of surgically treated thyroid cancer in children of Belarus. Ann. Surg. 243 (4), 525–532. Available from: http://dx.doi.org/10.1097/01.sla.0000205977.74806.0b.

Fridman, M., Demidchik, Y., Drozd, V., Reiners, C., 2016. Concerns about the American Thyroid Association Guidelines on Pediatric Thyroid Cancer. US Endocrinol. 12 (1), 24–25.

Fridman, M., Drozd, V., Demidchik, Y., Levin, L., Branovan, D., Shiglik, N., et al., 2015b. Second primary malignancies in Belarus patients with post-Chernobyl papillary thyroid carcinoma. Thyroid 25 (S1), A22–23.

Fridman, M., Lam, A.K., Krasko, O., 2016. Characteristics of young adults of Belarus with post-Chernobyl papillary thyroid carcinoma: a long-term follow-up of patients with early exposure to radiation at the 30th anniversary of the accident. Clin. Endocrinol. 85, 971–978.

Fridman, M., Lam, A.K., Krasko, O., Schmid, K.W., Branovan, D.I., Demidchik, Y., 2015a. Morphological and clinical presentation of papillary thyroid carcinoma in children and adolescents of Belarus: the influence of radiation exposure and the source of irradiation. Exp. Mol. Pathol. 98 (3), 527–531. Available from: http://dx.doi.org/10.1016/j.yexmp.2015.03.039.

Fridman, M., Savva, N., Krasko, O., Mankovskaya, S., Branovan, D.I., Schmid, K.W., et al., 2014. Initial presentation and late results of treatment of post-Chernobyl papillary thyroid carcinoma in children and adolescents of Belarus. J. Clin. Endocrinol. Metab. 99 (8), 2932–2941. Available from: http://dx.doi.org/10.1210/jc.2013-3131.

Kenigsberg, Y., Buglova, E., Kruk, J., Golovneva, A., 2002. Ehyroid cancer among children and adolescents of Belarus exposed due to the Chernobyl accident: Dose and risk assessment. In: Yamashita, S., Shibata, Y., Hoshi, M., Fujimura, K. (Eds.), Chernobyl: Message for the 21st Century. Elsevier, Amsterdam, pp. 293–300.

Nikiforov, Y.E., 2002. RET/PTC rearrangement in thyroid tumors. Endocr. Pathol. 13 (1), 3–16.

Rumyantsev, P.O., Saenko, V.A., Ilyin, A.A., Stepanenko, V.F., Rumyantseva, U.V., Abrosimov, A.Y., et al., 2011. Radiation exposure does not significantly contribute to the risk of recurrence of Chernobyl thyroid cancer. J. Clin. Endocrinol. Metab. 96 (2), 385–393. Available from: http://dx.doi.org/10.1210/jc.2010-1634.

Thomas, G.A., Bunnell, H., Cook, H.A., Williams, E.D., Nerovnya, A., Cherstvoy, E.D., et al., 1999. High prevalence of RET/PTC rearrangements in Ukrainian and Belarussian post-Chernobyl thyroid papillary carcinomas: a strong correlation between RET/PTC3 and the solid-follicular variant. J. Clin. Endocrinol. Metab. 84 (11), 4232–4238. Available from: http://dx.doi.org/10.1210/jcem.84.11.6129.

CHAPTER 6

Clinical Aspects of Pediatric Thyroid Cancer and Follow-Up of Patients in Belarus Following the Chernobyl Accident

Valentina M. Drozd[1,2], Mikhail V. Fridman[3,7], Vladimir A. Saenko[4], Yuri E. Demidchik[2,7], Tamara Platonova[1], Igor Branovan[5], Nikolay Shiglik[5], Tatiana I. Rogounovitch[4], Shunichi Yamashita[4], Johannes Biko[6] and Christoph Reiners[6]

[1]The International Fund "Help for Patients with Radiation-Induced Thyroid Cancer "Arnica", Minsk, Belarus [2]Belarusian Medical Academy of Postgraduate Education, Minsk, Belarus [3]Minsk Municipal Clinical Oncological Dispensary, Minsk, Belarus [4]Nagasaki University, Nagasaki, Japan [5]Project Chernobyl, Brooklyn, NY, United States [6]University of Würzburg, Würzburg, Germany [7]Republican Centre for Thyroid Tumors, Minsk, Belarus

The incidence of pediatric thyroid cancer in Belarus increased dramatically during the years 1990—2005, as soon as 4 years after the Chernobyl accident. The role of radiation in thyroid cancer induction is now well proven. The influence of other factors, modifiers, and cofounders such as genetic predisposition, ecological pollutants, iodine deficiency, and their combined effects requires further investigation.

The first report of Belarusian doctors about an increased frequency of the number of thyroid cancer cases in children in Belarus was met with skepticism in Western countries, the US, and Japan. The comments by Shigematsu and Thiessen (1992) on the publication by Kazakov et al. (1992) were the following: the data provided in these reports are limited and preliminary in that they do not allow one to state whether the suggested increase in thyroid cancer cases is unequivocally attributable to radiation exposure because it included no information on screening data, control groups, and thyroid doses (Shigematsu and Thiessen, 1992). A later article by Williams (2006) stated that at that time "it was not thought plausible that exposure to radio-isotopes of iodine in fallout could lead to such an increase in thyroid cancer with such a short latency."

Thyroid Cancer and Nuclear Accidents. DOI: http://dx.doi.org/10.1016/B978-0-12-812768-1.00006-X

In retrospect, the skepticism was unjustified. In 1996, 4 years after the first report, the IAEA admitted that the increased incidence of thyroid cancer in children was caused by Chernobyl radiation: "A sharp increase in thyroid cancer among children from the affected areas is the only major public health impact from radiation exposure documented to date" ("Ten Years After Chernobyl: What Do We Really Know?", 1996). The article by the Belarusian scientists also pointed out that tumors detected in children before 1992 had aggressive behavior (Furmanchuk et al., 1992). Extrathyroidal extension was observed in 60.5%, regional lymph node metastases in 74%, and distant metastases in 7%. Clinical and morphological comparisons in ultrasound diagnosis of carcinoma in children exposed to radiation have shown that the diffuse sclerosing variant of papillary thyroid carcinoma (PTC) occurred more frequently in patients with higher doses to the thyroid. This variant of PTC was rarely found at pT1 stage and was more frequently accompanied by bilateral and mediastinal metastases than typical and follicular variant of PC (Cherstvoj et al., 1996). Modern molecular studies of post-Chernobyl thyroid cancer showed that *RET/PTC3* is linked to a more aggressive behavior than *RET/PTC1* and *BRAF* mutations. *RET/PTC3* is related to the solid variant of PTC, while *RET/PTC1* is more frequent than typical papillary tumors (Nikiforov et al., 1997; Rabes et al., 2000). Studies of radiation-induced thyroid cancer in Belarus after the Chernobyl accident demonstrated that radiation dose was significantly associated with thyroid cancer incidence. Furthermore, the effect of radiation displayed regional variations according to nitrate concentration in drinking water (Drozd et al., 2015).

The aim of the current study was to evaluate factors modifying risk for and to analyze clinical aspects of radiation-induced PTC in the Belarusian pediatric population after the Chernobyl accident.

METHOD

Patients

The prevalence of pediatric thyroid cancer in rural/urban areas, pathological and clinical characteristics were investigated among 1078 children and adolescents (61.9% female, 38.1% male) with PTC, who were surgically treated from 1990 to 2005. Mean age ($\pm$ SD) of patients at surgery was 13 ($\pm$ 3.5) years. The median follow-up was 15.4 years.

RESULTS

The crude prevalence of the pediatric thyroid cancer population for the period of time from 1990 to 2005 in rural/urban areas of different oblasts (an administrative equivalent of a state or prefecture) of Belarus was as follows: Gomel 408/168, Brest 181/76, Mogilev 70/21, Minsk 25/25, Grodno 28/32, Vitebsk 7/13. A significantly higher ($P < 0.001$) prevalence of thyroid cancer among rural residents as compared with urban was found in Gomel, Mogilev, and Brest Oblasts with higher thyroid doses. In contrast, there was no difference in the prevalence of thyroid cancer in three other oblasts of Minsk, Grodno, and Vitebsk, where thyroid doses were substantially lower (see Fig. 6.1).

The level of nitrate in drinking water was especially high at the beginning of the 1990s in rural areas of Gomel and Brest Oblasts, exceeding the WHO's recommended maximum contaminant level 2.5- and 4.0-fold, respectively, while in Mogilev it was in the normal range. Average concentration of nitrates in open wells water in the early 1990s were in Gomel 112, Mogilev 40, and Brest 185 mg/L. The proportion of thyroid cancer was significantly higher in Gomel Oblast, in comparison with Brest and Mogilev ($P < 0.05$), for both rural and urban residents, which can be explained by the higher average doses to

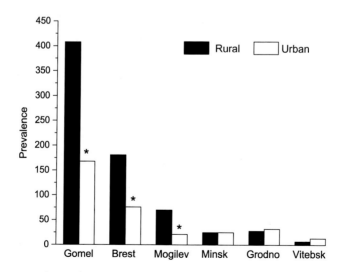

*Figure 6.1 Cumulative prevalence of thyroid cancer in children and adolescents in 1986–2005 by rural/urban type of settlement of residence. Names of oblasts are indicated under the horizontal axis. *Significant difference between the prevalence of thyroid cancer in pediatric population residing in rural and urban settlements (P < 0.001).*

the thyroid in this oblast (320 mGy). Mean thyroid doses in Brest and Mogilev oblasts were about the same (Mogilev 65, and Brest 51 mGy), however the proportion of thyroid cancer in Brest was significantly higher than in Mogilev ($P < 0.05$). We hypothesize that a higher concentration of nitrates in drinking water of Brest Oblast may be linked to these discrepancies. Rural residents at the time of Chernobyl accident might have been at higher risk for thyroid cancer not only because of the higher I-131 doses received by the thyroid, but also due to exposure to other modifying factors including consumption of drinking water with high nitrate content (Drozd et al., 2016).

Early diagnosis of thyroid cancer in children exposed to radionuclides is a very important clinical aspect of a good outcome. We analyzed ultrasound features of thyroid cancer in children to find typical echo-symptoms. According to our experience, ultrasonic patterns of thyroid cancer in childhood patients exposed to radionuclides could be nodular and diffuse. The nodular pattern can be subdivided into nodules with the confined spread (with regular margins), and nodules with undetermined spread (with irregular margins). The diffuse variant is characterized by essential volume enlargement of the thyroid (usually more than two times) with a diffuse structure modification, hypo- or mixed, inhomogeneous echogenicity. We observed the diffuse pattern only from 1990 to 1995 in 7% of patients 8–15 years old with the short latent period. More frequently, the tumor is visualized as a hypoechoic nodule (62%) with inhomogeneous structure (84%) and irregular outline (63%), with enlarged regional lymph nodes (66%). The most straightforward ultrasonic evidence of cancer is enlarged isoechoic regional lymph nodes, which are rounded and often form packs (Drozd et al., 1993, 2002, 2009).

Fine-needle aspiration (FNA) biopsy of thyroid nodular lesions is a safe procedure that does not cause significant changes to volumes or the structure of nodular lesions. Only in 1% of cases did we observe local change of echogenicity which can be interpreted as a small hemorrhage induced by FNA. Performing FNA regardless of the size of the nodule, once indicated or accessible, could promote early diagnosis of thyroid cancer in young subjects with a history of radiation exposure.

The analysis of long-term treatment results of 1078 children and adolescents who were surgically treated from 1990 to 2005 showed a rather favorable outcome. The overall survival was 96.9% with a median follow-up of 15.4 years. Total thyroidectomy (TT) (68.6%) and radioactive iodine therapy (62.7%) were the most frequent treatment modalities. The 20-year event-free survival was 87.8%. The type of surgery (TT vs. non-TT) influenced the cumulative incidence of both locoregional and distant relapses of PTC in exposed children. Relapse-free survival after TT at 5, 10, and 20 years was $97.8\% \pm 0.6\%$, $97.0\% \pm 0.7\%$, and $97.0\% \pm 0.7\%$, respectively. For comparison, relapse-free survival after non-TT at 5, 10, and 20 years was $92.8\% \pm 1.5\%$, $88.3\% \pm 1.9\%$, and $84.5\% \pm 2.2\%$, respectively (Fridman et al., 2014).

Pathomorphological analysis indicates that pediatric patients had a high rate of metastatic PTC at presentation: 73.8% lymph nodes involvement, 11.1% distant metastasis, 41.3% extrathyroidal extent, 6.4% multifocality, 18.8% blood and 84.4% lymphatic vessel invasion. The average tumor size was 14.4 mm (range $1-124$ mm). Classical PTC was observed in 38.5%, follicular variant in 31.2%, diffuse sclerosing in 7.8%, tall cell in 6.9%, clear cell in 1.1%, and solid in 14.5% cases (Fridman et al., 2014).

Patients in the younger age group, as compared with older children and adolescents, more frequently had locally advanced disease (N1) and distant metastases (M1) ($P < 0.001$). The strongest factor for extrathyroidal extension was infiltrative growth or diffuse intrathyroidal spread (OR = 9.48, 95% CI = $3.50-30.73$), for lymph node metastases/lymphatic vessel invasion (OR = 23.41, 95% CI = $11.66-50.84$), and for distant metastases/lateral lymph node involvement (OR = 6.08, 95% CI = $3.43-11.31$).

During the period from 1991 through 2014, among 1078 patients diagnosed for thyroid cancer in childhood or adolescent age, 15 (1.4%) developed second primary malignancy (SPM), and 21 (1.9%) patients died. Only two patients died due to thyroid cancer or cancer-related post-therapeutic complications (advanced disease and pulmonary fibrosis, respectively). Other deaths were due to SPM (gastric adenocarcinoma, two cases of acute lymphoblastic leukemia; three patients), seven patients committed suicide, six died due to accidents/traumas, and three patients died due to acute cardiac failure and liver cirrhosis (Fridman et al., 2014).

Among 15 individuals with SPM, solid cancers were detected in 10 patients (66.7%): breast cancer (one), basal cell carcinoma (one), melanoma (two); female genital system (two: cervical cancer in situ (one), vulvar cancer (one)), the alimentary tract (three: colon cancer (Gardner syndrome) [one], gastric cancer (one), parotid gland mucoepidermoid carcinoma (one)). One patient developed malignant schwannoma. Five hematological malignancies were registered: acute leukemia (three), non-Hodgkin lymphoma (one), and Hodgkin's lymphoma (one).

DISCUSSION

Our study demonstrates a relatively good prognosis in children and adolescents diagnosed with thyroid cancer regardless of the aggressive presentation once early diagnosis and appropriate therapy have been performed. More frequently, the post-Chernobyl radiogenic PTC in young patients is visualized by ultrasound as a hypoechoic node with inhomogeneous structure and irregular outline with enlarged regional lymph nodes, however some cases may have a diffuse form. Despite tumor size usually being moderate, nodal disease is frequent, and distant metastases were observed in approximately one in 10 patients. Even when a disease is advanced and initially suboptimally treated, outcomes are generally favorable after TT and radioiodine therapy, which are the most common treatment modalities. The prevalence of SPM in the unique cohort of young adults treated for post-Chernobyl PTC at pediatric age is 1.4%. Fatalities during 1991–2014 were rare (1.9%), and suicide and trauma were the most frequent causes of death, indicating a need for improvement of psychological rehabilitation. Future research and follow-up are important to evaluate the impact of irradiation (from Chernobyl and therapeutic), genetic predisposition, and environment factors in determining the long-term outcomes of pediatric thyroid cancer.

REFERENCES

Cherstvoj, E.D., Demidchik, E.P., & Drozd, V.M. (1996, April). *Clinico-morphological comparisons in ultrasound diagnosis of carcinoma of the thyroid in children exposed to radiation.* Poster session presented at the One decade after Chernobyl. Summing up the consequences of the accident, Vienna.

Drozd, V.M., Astakhova, L.N., Polyanskaya, O.N., Kobzev, V.F., Nalivko, A.S., & Tolkachev, Y.V. (1993). *Ultrasonic diagnostics of thyroid pathology in children and adolescents effected by radionuclides.* Paper presented at the International Congress on Interventional Ultrasound, Copenhagen.

Drozd, V., Fridman, M., Brenner, A., Drozdovitch, V., Platonova, T., Branovan, I., et al. (2016, October). Comparison of the prevalence of radiation induced childhood thyroid cancer in rural and urban populations of Belarus after the Chernobyl accident. Paper presented at the 62nd Annual International Meeting of the Radiation Research Society, Big Island, HI.

Drozd, V.M., Lushchik, M.L., Polyanskaya, O.N., Fridman, M.V., Demidchik, Y.E., Lyshchik, A.P., et al., 2009. The usual ultrasonographic features of thyroid cancer are less frequent in small tumors that develop after a long latent period after the Chernobyl radiation release accident. Thyroid 19 (7), 725−734. Available from: http://dx.doi.org/10.1089/thy.2008.0238.

Drozd, V., Polyanskaya, O., Ostapenko, V., Demidchik, Y., Biko, I., Reiners, C., 2002. Systematic ultrasound screening as a significant tool for early detection of thyroid carcinoma in Belarus. J. Pediatr. Endocrinol. Metab. 15 (7), 979−984.

Drozd, V.M., Saenko, V.A., Brenner, A.V., Drozdovitch, V., Pashkevich, V.I., Kudelsky, A.V., et al., 2015. Major factors affecting incidence of childhood thyroid cancer in Belarus after the Chernobyl accident: do nitrates in drinking water play a role? PLoS One 10 (9), e0137226. Available from: http://dx.doi.org/10.1371/journal.pone.0137226.

Fridman, M., Savva, N., Krasko, O., Mankovskaya, S., Branovan, D.I., Schmid, K.W., et al., 2014. Initial presentation and late results of treatment of post-Chernobyl papillary thyroid carcinoma in children and adolescents of Belarus. J. Clin. Endocrinol. Metab. 99 (8), 2932−2941. Available from: http://dx.doi.org/10.1210/jc.2013-3131.

Furmanchuk, A.W., Averkin, J.I., Egloff, B., Ruchti, C., Abelin, T., Schappi, W., et al., 1992. Pathomorphological findings in thyroid cancers of children from the Republic of Belarus: a study of 86 cases occurring between 1986 ('post-Chernobyl') and 1991. Histopathology 21 (5), 401−408.

Kazakov, V.S., Demidchik, E.P., Astakhova, L.N., 1992. Thyroid cancer after Chernobyl. Nature 359 (6390), 21. Available from: http://dx.doi.org/10.1038/359021a0.

Nikiforov, Y.E., Rowland, J.M., Bove, K.E., Monforte-Munoz, H., Fagin, J.A., 1997. Distinct pattern of ret oncogene rearrangements in morphological variants of radiation-induced and sporadic thyroid papillary carcinomas in children. Cancer Res. 57 (9), 1690−1694.

Rabes, H.M., Demidchik, E.P., Sidorow, J.D., Lengfelder, E., Beimfohr, C., Hoelzel, D., et al., 2000. Pattern of radiation-induced RET and NTRK1 rearrangements in 191 post-chernobyl papillary thyroid carcinomas: biological, phenotypic, and clinical implications. Clin. Cancer Res. 6 (3), 1093−1103.

Shigematsu, I., Thiessen, J.W., 1992. Comment on childhood thyroid cancer in Belarus. Nature 359 (6397), 681.

Ten Years After Chernobyl: What Do We Really Know? Based on the proceedings of the IAEA/WHO/EC International Conference, Vienna, April 1996. (1996). International Atomic Energy Agency, Vienna, Austria: Division of Public Information.

Williams, E.D., 2006. Chernobyl and thyroid cancer. J. Surg. Oncol. 94 (8), 670−677. Available from: http://dx.doi.org/10.1002/jso.20699.

CHAPTER 7

Long-Term Analysis of the Incidence and Histopathology of Thyroid Cancer in Ukraine in Adult Patients Who Were Children and Adolescents at the Time of the Chernobyl Accident

Tetiana Bogdanova[1], Vladimir A. Saenko[2], Victor Shpak[1],
Liudmyla Zurnadzhy[1], Laryssa Voskoboynyk[1], Tetiana Dekhtyarova[1],
Svitlana Burko[1], Tamara Gulii[1], Shunichi Yamashita[2] and
Mykola Tronko[1]

[1]V.P. Komisarenko Institute of Endocrinology and Metabolism of National Academy of Medical Sciences of Ukraine, Kyiv, Ukraine [2]Nagasaki University, Nagasaki, Japan

An increase in thyroid cancer incidence in the affected population of Belarus, Ukraine, and the Russian Federation is a major scientifically proven and generally accepted by the international community health effect of the Chernobyl disaster, which occurred in Ukraine on April 26, 1986. The specific temporal and geographic distribution of thyroid cancer cases diagnosed in young patients was suggestive of a common causative event. It was unambiguously established later that the internal exposure of the thyroid gland to radioiodine was the cause. Thyroid dose per unit of ingested iodine isotope is higher for children than for adults, mostly due to the smaller size of the thyroid in children. That is why the group at higher risk for developing radiogenic thyroid cancer includes individuals who had experienced exposure to radioactive fallout in their childhood and adolescence (Jacob et al., 2006; Saenko et al., 2011; Tronko et al., 2010, 2014).

A number of studies have addressed the morphological characteristics of thyroid cancer, especially of the papillary thyroid carcinomas (PTC) detected in children and adolescents at the time of the surgery (Bogdanova et al., 2014; Fridman et al., 2015; LiVolsi et al., 2011; Williams et al., 2004). As it is now 30 years since the Chernobyl

Thyroid Cancer and Nuclear Accidents. DOI: http://dx.doi.org/10.1016/B978-0-12-812768-1.00007-1

accident, and those exposed during childhood and adolescence have become adults, it is therefore important to clarify the changes to pathological characteristics over time in this exposed population.

Tumor-invasive properties occupy a special place in the histopathological analysis of post-Chernobyl papillary carcinomas. Factors such as extrathyroidal extension and regional lymph node involvement strongly affect the treatment strategy and the chance of recurrence in the postoperative period (Nikiforov et al., 2012; Rosai, 2011). In addition, histopathological analysis of PTCs detected during screening of specific cohorts established an association between invasive properties of PTC and thyroid radiation dose: linear in the Belarusian cohort (Zablotska et al., 2015) and linear-quadratic in the Ukrainian one (Bogdanova et al., 2015). At present, definitive conclusions about changes in the invasive properties of post-Chernobyl PTC are available for patients operated on during their childhood and adolescence (Bogdanova et al., 2014; Fridman et al., 2015), no new cases in these age groups naturally exist from 2001 and 2005, respectively. However, morphological studies of PTC in adults belonging to the high-risk group (i.e., those exposed at the age of 0–18 years old) should continue. In this regard, this chapter focuses on the incidence and histopathological characteristics of thyroid carcinomas through a long period of time after the accident (up to 28 years) only in the group of Ukrainian adults aged from 19 to 46 years at the time of surgery.

METHODS
Subjects and Sources of Data
The Clinical-Morphological Registry (CMR) of thyroid cancer in subjects of high-risk group was established in V.P. Komisarenko Institute of Endocrinology and Metabolism of the National Academy of Medical Sciences of Ukraine (IEM) in 1992 and is maintained until the present day. All cases of thyroid cancer in patients whose age at the time of the accident did not exceed 18 years (i.e., born in 1968 and later) are registered. The CMR is a specialized registry that includes patients of that particular age group and only operated cases with pathologically confirmed diagnosis. Pathological verification of diagnosis is essential for any case to be included in the CMR. The detailed pathological report including tumor type, subtype, invasive properties, and tumor size is mandatory for cases

operated at the Department of Surgery of Endocrine Glands of the IEM, and for the patients operated elsewhere in Ukraine but receiving radioiodine therapy at the Department of Clinical Radiology of the IEM. Sources of information for the CMR are currently the reports of regional endocrinology services, data of regional oncology institutions (via the National cancer registry of Ukraine), and clinical medical information system of the IEM.

To calculate the incidence, the most adequate determination of the number of person-years in a given cohort for a particular year is to use the average population size. For the current analysis, adult cases (aged ≥19 years at surgery, and born before the Chernobyl accident in 1968–1985) have been selected from the CMR, and a classification of 28 regions of Ukraine into two groups according to the level of thyroid exposure was used (Likhtarov et al., 2014):

1. The six most contaminated regions (Zhytomyr, Kyiv, Rivne, Chernihiv, Cherkasy regions, and Kyiv City; average thyroid exposure dose in the group 0–18 years old at the time of the accident >35 mGy); and
2. Twenty-one regions with relatively lower levels of contamination (average thyroid exposure dose in the group 0–18 years old <35 mGy).

The period of study was from 1986 to 2014 (preliminary data for 2014 do not include information for Donetsk and Luhansk oblasts, and Sevastopol city) due to recent political changes in Ukraine.

Histopathological Analysis
Histopathological analysis included 2634 thyroid cancer cases registered during 2002–05, 2006–08, 2009–11, and 2012–14 in patients aged from 19 to 46 years. The histological type of thyroid carcinoma was classified according to the World Health Organization classification (DeLellis et al., 2004). Most cases have been additionally verified by a panel of experts/pathologists of the Chernobyl Tissue Bank (Thomas and Williams, 2000). The diagnosis of thyroid carcinoma was confirmed in all these cases. Tumor stage was characterized according to the 7th edition of the TNM classification system (Sobin et al., 2010), which classified the minimal extrathyroidal extension as pT3 category (Su et al., 2016). Distant metastases to the lungs were determined by radioactive iodine scans performed following thyroidectomy.

Statistical Analysis

Calculations were performed with the InStat package (GraphPad software, Inc., La Jolla, CA, USA). Comparisons for count data performed using the Fisher exact test and the Cochran-Armitage test were run to assess a linear trend.

RESULTS

The interpretation of the number of cases and incidence in the groups defined by the age at surgery should take into account that the composition of such groups changes from year to year as the cohorts become older. In the age group of ≥ 19 years old at surgery, incidence trends were markedly different from the younger groups described in our previous publication (Tronko et al., 2014). This group has no upper age limit, and its size, median age, and age structure changes every year. Incidence rates in the six and 21 regions show increasing trends. At the same time, the incidence rate in the six most contaminated regions exceeded that in the 21 low-contaminated regions more than twofold during the period from 1998 to 2014 (Table 7.1).

Pathological analysis showed that the PTC prevailed in every period under study (92.7% overall). Follicular carcinoma was diagnosed in 5.2%, medullary carcinoma in 1.7%, and poorly differentiated carcinoma in only 0.4% of all cases (Table 7.2).

Distribution of the frequency of fully encapsulated tumors, tumor size, dominant pattern, and the main histological characteristics that reflect their invasiveness, including extrathyroidal extension, regional, and distant metastases are presented in Table 7.3.

Histopathological characteristics of PTC significantly changed over time after Chernobyl, i.e., with latency. Two linear time trends (increasing and decreasing) were revealed for most pathological characteristics under study. Increasing linear trends were found for the frequencies of fully encapsulated tumors and the so-called "small' tumors sized ≤ 10 mm. Significant changes were observed in the structural characteristics of PTCs: frequency of the tumors with dominant solid pattern (DSP) linearly decreased with time, and frequency of the tumors with dominant papillary pattern (DPP), on the contrary, increased with time. The frequency of PTCs with dominant follicular pattern (DFP) did not undergo substantial changes with time since the accident.

Table 7.1 Thyroid Cancer Cases and Incidence Per 100,000 in Subjects Aged ≥19 at Surgery (≤18 at the Time of the Chernobyl Accident)

	1986	1987	1988	1989	1990	1991	1992	1993	1994	1995	1996	1997	1998	1999	2000	2001	2002	2003	2004	2005	2006	2007	2008	2009	2010	2011	2012	2013	2014
Cases (F)	0	2	3	4	19	19	33	55	65	91	83	114	145	166	165	255	248	234	300	339	402	435	514	538	574	766	740	836	806
Cases (M)	0	0	1	4	2	7	12	13	9	17	21	26	23	41	34	53	59	55	50	73	85	92	98	100	133	137	144	177	165
Cases (both)	0	2	4	8	21	26	45	68	74	108	104	140	168	207	199	308	307	289	350	412	487	527	612	638	707	903	884	1013	971
Incidence	–	0.6	0.4	0.5	0.9	0.8	1.2	1.4	1.5	1.8	1.5	1.9	2.1	2.3	2.1	2.9	2.7	2.4	2.8	3.1	3.7	4.0	4.6	4.8	5.2	6.7	6.5	7.5	7.2
6 Regions, cases (both)	0	1	0	3	5	10	13	16	16	39	33	35	67	80	88	134	133	120	140	160	210	214	230	252	259	330	307	358	369
21 Regions, cases (both)	0	1	4	5	16	16	32	52	58	69	71	105	101	127	111	174	174	169	210	252	277	313	382	386	448	573	577	655	602
6 Regions, incidence	–	1.5	–	0.9	1.1	1.6	1.7	1.6	1.5	3.2	2.4	2.5	4.1	4.5	4.5	6.4	6.0	5.0	5.5	6.0	7.8	8.0	8.5	9.3	9.6	12.1	11.4	13.3	13.2
21 Regions, incidence	–	0.4	0.5	0.4	0.9	0.7	1	1.4	1.4	1.4	1.3	1.7	1.6	1.8	1.4	2.1	1.9	1.8	2.1	2.4	2.6	2.9	3.6	3.6	4.2	5.3	5.3	6.1	5.7

Table 7.2 Types of Thyroid Carcinoma Detected in Ukrainian Patients Aged ≥19 years at Surgery (≤18 years at the Time of the Chernobyl Accident)

Tumor type	2002–2005 (n = 511)		2006–2008 (n = 640)		2009–2011 (n = 727)		2012–2014 (n = 756)		2002–2014 (n = 2634)	
	Number	%	Number	%	Number	%	Number	%	Number	%
Papillary	465	91.0	584	91.2	2442	92.7	705	93.3	2442	92.7
Follicular	35	6.8	41	6.4	136	5.2	34	4.5	136	5.2
Medullary	8	1.6	13	2.0	46	1.7	14	1.8	46	1.7
Poorly differentiated	3	0.6	2	0.4	10	0.4	3	0.4	10	0.4
Anaplastic	0	0	0	0	0	0	0	0	0	0

Table 7.3 Characteristics of the Papillary Thyroid Carcinoma Detected in Ukrainian Patients Aged ≥ 19 years at Surgery (≤18 years at the Time of the Chernobyl Accident)

	All cases								
	2002–2005 (n = 465)		2006–2008 (n = 584)		2009–2011 (n = 688)		2012–2014 (n = 705)		P-value
	Number	%	Number	%	Number	%	Number	%	for trend
Capsule									
Full	96	20.6	130	22.3	184	26.7	192	27.2	0.003
Partial/absent	369	79.4	454	77.7	504	73.3	513	72.8	
Size									
≤ 10 mm	97	20.9	152	26.0	273	39.7	307	43.6	<0.0001
>10 mm	368	79.1	432	74.0	415	60.3	398	56.4	
Dominant Pattern									
Papillary	232	49.9	293	50.2	358	52.0	390	55.3	0.042
Follicular	137	29.5	176	30.1	210	30.6	222	31.5	0.447
Solid-trabecular	96	20.6	115	19.7	120	17.4	93	13.2	0.0003
Invasiveness									
Extrathyroidal extension (T3)	128	27.5	153	26.2	154	22.4	142	20.1	0.0009
Multifocality (Tm)	32	6.9	72	12.3	143	20.8	154	21.8	<0.0001
Lymph node metastases (N1)	148	31.8	168	28.8	185	26.9	208	29.5	0.751
Distant metastases (M1)	18	3.9	11	1.9	9	1.3	10	1.4	0.005
Concomitant Pathology									
Nodular	43	9.3	78	13.4	152	22.1	183	26.0	<0.0001
Diffuse	82	17.6	114	19.5	208	30.2	193	27.4	<0.0001
Chronic thyroiditis	78	16.8	102	17.5	176	25.6	180	25.5	<0.0001

In the last period of observation (2012–14), the percentage of PTCs with DPP was 4.2 times higher than that with DSP ($P < 0.0001$; OR = 8.141). Meanwhile, the proportion of fully encapsulated tumors among PTCs with DPP was 4.8 times lower than in tumors with DSP (48/390 or 12.3% vs. 55/93 or 59.1%; $P < 0.0001$; OR = 0.097).

It should also be noted that during the last period of observation, PTCs with DPP were characterized by the more pronounced invasive properties as compared with tumors with DFP, and especially with DSP. Extrathyroidal extension and regional metastases were detected in PTC with DPP in 22.8% (89/390 cases) and in 37.9% (148/390 cases), respectively. In tumors with DFP these were 18.4% (41/222 cases, $P = 0.219$ vs. PTC with DPP) and in 20.7% (46/222 cases, $P < 0.0001$ vs. PTC with DPP), and for PTC with DSP in 12.9% (12/93 cases, $P = 0.034$ vs. PTC with DPP) and 15.1% (14/93 cases, $P < 0.0001$ vs. PTC with DPP), respectively.

In general, the invasiveness of PTCs in terms of extrathyroidal extension and distant lung metastases significantly decreased with increasing time after the accident, but no significant changes in the frequency of regional lymph node metastases were observed. An increasing linear time trend was observed for multifocal or multiple PTCs. Concomitant benign thyroid pathology, both nodular and diffuse (mainly chronic thyroiditis) also showed the increasing time trends over time (see Table 7.3).

DISCUSSION

In the previous studies of Ukrainian pediatric post-Chernobyl thyroid cancer, the so-called "childhood" variant, which combines nonencapsulated PTC with solid and solid-follicular patterns, and especially tumors with a shorter period of latency (during the first decade after Chernobyl), displayed the most aggressive biological behavior (Bogdanova et al., 2014; LiVolsi et al., 2011; Williams et al., 2004). In contrast, PTC with DSP in adults aged 26–46 years and operated in 2012–14 after 26–28 years of latency was characterized by the highest frequency of fully encapsulated tumors. Such tumors do not commonly feature extrathyroidal extension and lymph node metastases indicative of their limited invasiveness. The more pronounced invasive properties were noted among PTCs with DPP, which were characterized by the higher frequencies of nonencapsulated tumors, extrathyroidal extension, and the presence of lymph node metastases.

Regarding the increase in the percentage of microcarcinoma to 43.6%, this is in line with the suggestion that this is due in part to the improvement in ultrasound equipment and fine-needle aspiration biopsy technique (Leboulleux, et al., 2016). However, in our studies, micro-PTCs sized ≤ 10 mm showed signs of extrathyroidal extension in 13.4% (41/307 cases), lymph node involvement in 19.5% (60/307 cases), and distant metastases to the lung in 0.3% (1/307 cases).

This demonstrates that small tumors require careful attention and thorough evaluation regarding the treatment in each individual case.

In conclusion, our study demonstrates that significantly increased thyroid cancer incidence in the residents of Ukraine who were children and adolescents at the time of the Chernobyl accident, but reached adulthood at the time of surgery, persists up to 2014, and the incidence rate in the six most contaminated regions by ^{131}I exceeded that in the 21 less contaminated regions.

Pathological analysis showed that PTC was the most prevalent type of thyroid cancer in all studied periods. In recent years, 43.6% PTCs measuring ≤ 10 mm was detected, which reflects the improvement of diagnostic methods. Almost one-third of all PTCs are fully encapsulated tumors with minimal invasive properties; a large proportion of them have dominant solid growth pattern. With increasing time after the accident, PTCs with a DPP exhibit more pronounced invasive properties, but in general PTCs clearly become less aggressive, which is an important favorable sign for the postoperative prognosis.

ACKNOWLEDGMENTS

We acknowledge the commitment of the Surgery Department of IEM, where most of the participants of the study were operated on. We also thank the International Pathology Panel of the Chernobyl Tissue Bank: Professors A. Abrosimov, T. Bogdanova, N. Dvinskikh, G. Fadda, J. Hunt, M. Ito, V. Livolsi, J. Rosai, and E.D. Williams for diagnosis verification.

REFERENCES

Bogdanova, T., Zurnadzhy, L., LiVolsi, V.A., Williams, E.D., Ito, M., Nakashima, M., et al., 2014. Thyroid cancer pathology in Ukraine after Chernobyl. In: Tronko, M., Bogdanova, T., Saenko, V., Thomas, G.A., Likhtarov, I., Yamashita, S. (Eds.), Thyroid Cancer in Ukraine after Chernobyl: Dosimetry, Epidemiology, Pathology, Molecular Biology. Nagasaki Association for Hibakushas' Medical Care, Nagasaki, pp. 65–108.

Bogdanova, T.I., Zurnadzhy, L.Y., Nikiforov, Y.E., Leeman-Neill, R.J., Tronko, M.D., Chanock, S., et al., 2015. Histopathological features of papillary thyroid carcinomas detected during four screening examinations of a Ukrainian-American cohort. Br. J. Cancer 113 (11), 1556–1564. Available from: http://dx.doi.org/10.1038/bjc.2015.372.

DeLellis, R.A., Lloyd, R.V., Heutz, P.U., Eng, C. (Eds.), 2004. Pathology and Genetics of Tumours of Endocrine Organs. IARC Press, Lyon.

Fridman, M., Lam, A.K., Krasko, O., Schmid, K.W., Branovan, D.I., Demidchik, Y., 2015. Morphological and clinical presentation of papillary thyroid carcinoma in children and adolescents of Belarus: the influence of radiation exposure and the source of irradiation. Exp. Mol. Pathol. 98 (3), 527–531. Available from: http://dx.doi.org/10.1016/j.yexmp.2015.03.039.

Jacob, P., Bogdanova, T.I., Buglova, E., Chepurniy, M., Demidchik, Y., Gavrilin, Y., et al., 2006. Thyroid cancer among Ukrainians and Belarusians who were children or adolescents at the time of the Chernobyl accident. J. Radiol. Prot. 26 (1), 51−67. Available from: http://dx.doi.org/ 10.1088/0952-4746/26/1/003.

Leboulleux, S., Tuttle, R.M., Pacini, F., Schlumberger, M., 2016. Papillary thyroid microcarcinoma: time to shift from surgery to active surveillance? Lancet Diabetes Endocrinol. 4 (11), 933−942, http://dx.doi.org/10.1016/S2213-8587(16)30180-2.

Likhtarov, I., Kovgan, L., Masiuk, S., Talerko, M., Chepurny, M., Ivanova, et al., 2014. Thyroid cancer study among Ukrainian children exposed to radiation after the Chornobyl accident: improved estimates of the thyroid doses to the cohort members. Health Phys. 106 (3), 370−396. Available from: http://dx.doi.org/10.1097/HP.0b013e31829f3096.

LiVolsi, V.A., Abrosimov, A.A., Bogdanova, T., Fadda, G., Hunt, J.L., Ito, M., et al., 2011. The Chernobyl thyroid cancer experience: pathology. Clin. Oncol. 23 (4), 261−267. Available from: http://dx.doi.org/10.1016/j.clon.2011.01.160.

Nikiforov, Y., Biddinger, P.W., Thompson, L.D.R., 2012. Diagnostic Pathology and Molecular Genetics of the Thyroid, second ed. Wolters Kluwer Health/Lippincott Williams & Wilkins, Philadelphia.

Rosai, J., 2011. Thyroid gland. In: tenth ed. Rosai, J. (Ed.), Rosai and Ackerman's Surgical Pathology, vol. 1. Mosby, Edinburgh; New York, pp. 487−564.

Saenko, V., Ivanov, V., Tsyb, A., Bogdanova, T., Tronko, M., Demidchik, Y., et al., 2011. The Chernobyl accident and its consequences. Clin. Oncol. 23 (4), 234−243. Available from: http://dx. doi.org/10.1016/j.clon.2011.01.502.

Sobin, L.H., Gospodarowicz, M.K., Wittekind, Ch, International Union against Cancer, 2010. TNM Classification of Malignant Tumours, seventh ed. Wiley-Blackwell, Chichester, West Sussex, UK; Hoboken, NJ.

Su, H.K., Wenig, B.M., Haser, G.C., Rowe, M.E., Asa, S.L., Baloch, Z., et al., 2016. Interobserver variation in the pathologic identification of minimal extrathyroidal extension in papillary thyroid carcinoma. Thyroid 26 (4), 512−517. Available from: http://dx.doi.org/10.1089/ thy.2015.0508.

Thomas, G.A., Williams, E.D., 2000. Thyroid tumor banks. Science 289 (5488), 2283.

Tronko, M., Bogdanova, T., Voskoboynyk, L., Zurnadzhy, L., Shpak, V., Gulak, L., 2010. Radiation induced thyroid cancer: fundamental and applied aspects. Exp. Oncol. 32 (3), 200−204.

Tronko, M., Shpak, V., Bogdanova, T., Saenko, V., Yamashita, S., 2014. Epidemiology of thyroid cancer in Ukraine after Chernobyl. In: Tronko, M., Bogdanova, T., Saenko, V., Thomas, G. A., Likhtarov, I., Yamashita, S. (Eds.), Thyroid Cancer in Ukraine After Chernobyl: Dosimetry, Epidemiology, Pathology, Molecular Biology. Nagasaki Association for Hibakushas' Medical Care, Nagasaki, pp. 39−64.

Williams, E.D., Abrosimov, A., Bogdanova, T., Demidchik, E.P., Ito, M., LiVolsi, V., et al., 2004. Thyroid carcinoma after Chernobyl: latent period, morphology and aggressiveness. Br. J. Cancer 90 (11), 2219−2224. Available from: http://dx.doi.org/10.1038/sj.bjc.6601860.

Zablotska, L.B., Nadyrov, E.A., Rozhko, A.V., Gong, Z., Polyanskaya, O.N., McConnell, R.J., et al., 2015. Analysis of thyroid malignant pathologic findings identified during 3 rounds of screening (1997-2008) of a cohort of children and adolescents from Belarus exposed to radioiodines after the Chernobyl accident. Cancer 121 (3), 457−466. Available from: http://dx.doi.org/ 10.1002/cncr.29073.

CHAPTER 8

Thyroid Cancer Risk in Ukraine Following the Chernobyl Accident (The Ukrainian–American Cohort Thyroid Study)

Mykola Tronko[1], Alina Brenner[2], Tetiana Bogdanova[1], Victor Shpak[1], Maureen Hatch[2], Ilya Likhtarev[3], Andre Bouville[2], Valeriy Oliynyk[1], Galyna Zamotayeva[1], Vladimir Drozdovitch[2], Liudmyla Zurnadzhy[1], Mark P. Little[2], Valeriy Tereshchenko[1], Stephen Chanock[2] and Kiyohiko Mabuchi[2]

[1]V.P. Komisarenko Institute of Endocrinology and Metabolism of National Academy of Medical Sciences of Ukraine, Kyiv, Ukraine [2]National Cancer Institute, Rockville, MD, United States [3]National Scientific Center of Radiation Medicine, Kyiv, Ukraine

INTRODUCTION

The 1986 accident at the Chernobyl (Chornobyl) nuclear power plant remains the most serious nuclear accident in history. Beginning 4 years after the accident, a sharp rise in the number of thyroid cancer cases was observed among individuals exposed as children in Ukraine, Belarus, and the Russian Federation (Goldman, 1997; Kazakov et al., 1992; Likhtarev et al., 1995a). These initial observations were followed by case–control and ecological studies (Astakhova et al., 1998; Jacob et al., 1998), which also found increased risk of thyroid cancer. The excess thyroid cancer cases were thought to be largely the result of the release of radioactive iodine (I-131) from the Chernobyl reactor. However, the estimates of radiation-related risk from these studies were uncertain due to the possible influence of unquantified detection bias from mass thyroid screening and uncertainties in doses estimated based on self-reported data on residential history and dietary patterns.

To overcome these problems, the US National Cancer Institute (NCI) in collaboration with the Ministry of Health of Ukraine initiated a long-term thyroid screening study of thyroid cancer and benign thyroid diseases among the younger exposed populations in areas of Ukraine most contaminated by the Chernobyl accident (Ukrainian–American, or

Thyroid Cancer and Nuclear Accidents. DOI: http://dx.doi.org/10.1016/B978-0-12-812768-1.00008-3

UkrAm, Study) (Stezhko et al., 2004; Tronko et al., 2006; Brenner et al., 2011; Little et al., 2014). A similar study was also begun in Belarus, known as the Belarusian–American (BelAm) study (Stezhko et al., 2004; Zablotska et al., 2011; Little et al., 2015). Two important features were standardized thyroid screening conducted irrespective of dose to ensure unbiased ascertainment of thyroid diseases and well-characterized I-131 thyroid dose estimates based on a model incorporating thyroid activity measurements obtained shortly after the accident, personal interview data on residential history, and consumption of milk and other contaminated foodstuffs, and radioecological parameters.

THE COHORT

A detailed description of the study design, population target groups, and methods has been published previously (Stezhko et al., 2004).

Within a few weeks after the accident, measurements of gamma radiation emitted by the thyroid (so-called direct thyroid measurements) were performed in Ukraine on approximately 150,000 subjects (Likhtarev et al., 1995b). The potential members of the cohort study were subjects born between April 26, 1968 and April 26, 1986 (the date of the accident), who received direct thyroid measurements from May to June 1986, and were residents of selected districts of Chernihiv, Zhytomyr, or Kyiv oblasts at the time of the accident. A subsample of 32,385 subjects was selected from this list of eligible subjects and was divided into three groups based on preliminary estimates of their thyroid dose. The subsample included all the subjects ($n = 8,752$) in the highest-dose group (≥ 1 Gy) and a randomly selected samples from two lower-dose groups (0–0.29 and 0.30–0.99 Gy, with 15,391 and 8,242 subjects, respectively). From April 1998 through December 2000, a variety of methods were used to track and invite the selected subjects to participate in the screening study. As a result, between 1998 and 2000, 13,243 (40.9%) individuals received a baseline thyroid screening examination.

Table 8.1 gives descriptive statistics on the UkrAm cohort at the time of the accident. Both genders are represented nearly equally (49% males and 51% females). Children aged 0–14 represent 94% of the cohort; only 6% of cohort members were 15–18 years old at the time of the accident. At that time, cohort members were more likely to be

Table 8.1 Basic Characteristics of the UkrAm Thyroid Cohort at the Time of the Accident (*n* = 13,243)

	n	%
Gender		
Male	6514	49
Female	6729	51
Age on April 26, 1986 (years)		
0–4	4531	34
5–9	3936	30
10–14	3961	30
≥ 15	815	6
Oblast Residence in 1986		
Chernihiv	6959	52
Kyiv	2600	20
Zhytomyr	3684	28
Urban Status in 1986		
Urban	4752	36
Rural	8491	64
Distance From Chernobyl NPP		
< 30 km	1247	9
30–59.9 km	1834	14
60–99.9 km	8478	64
≥ 100 km	1684	13

residents of rural areas (64%). The residents of the 30 km zone (9%) (town of Pripyat and Chernobyl district) were immediately evacuated within the first days of the accident. The majority of cohort members (64%) resided within 60–100 km of the damaged Chernobyl reactor. At the time of the first screening almost all members of the cohort lived in Chernihiv, Kyiv, Zhytomyr regions, and in Kyiv City.

SCREENING PROCEDURES

The standardized medical screening procedures were described in Tronko et al. (2006) and Brenner et al. (2011). Patients who had thyroid nodules detected by ultrasonography that measured at least 10 mm and all nodules that measured 5–9 mm and were sonographically suspicious for malignancy (hypoechogenic, indistinct border, calcified inclusions, extension through the thyroid capsule, or suspicious lymphadenopathy) were referred to the Clinical Department of the Institute of Endocrinology (Kyiv) for ultrasound-guided fine needle aspiration (FNA) biopsy. The patients were referred for surgery if, on cytology, the lesion was either suspicious for, or confirmed to be, thyroid cancer or follicular neoplasm.

The study pathologists diagnosed thyroid cancers based on examination of tumor tissue. All diagnoses were confirmed by an International Pathology Panel of the Chernobyl Tissue Bank (CTB) (Bogdanova et al., 2015).

Following the first screening examination in 1998–2000, the cohort members were screened three times (every 2 years) during 2001–07 according to a standardized protocol. After the fourth cycle of screening, those with previously identified nodular pathology had additional screening examinations through 2012 ("Nodular Project"). For the rest of the cohort, thyroid and nonthyroid cancers were ascertained by passive follow-up through linkage with the National Cancer Registry. The fifth cycle of active screening was begun in 2012 and lasted until December 2015. Table 8.2 provides descriptive data on the screening rounds to date.

DOSIMETRY

Unlike many other studies of thyroid cancer in relation to environmental exposure post-Chernobyl thyroid dosimetry is based on an extended set of direct activity measurements (Likhtarev et al., 1995b; NCRP, 2008). The assessment of the individual thyroid doses due to intake of I-131 for

Table 8.2 Numbers of Cohort Members Examined in Each Screening Round and Numbers of Detected Thyroid Cancer Cases			
Screening Cycle	Calendar Years	Number of Examined Subjects and Response Rate	Detected Thyroid Cancer Cases
Before UkrAm screening	1990–1997	–	14[a]
First cycle	1998–2000	13,243 (100%)	45
Second cycle	2001–03	12,419 (94%)	32
Third cycle	2003–05	11,744 (89%)	17
Fourth cycle	2005–08	10,186 (77%)	16
Nodular project, passive screening	2009–11	–	22
Fifth cycle	2012–15	10,116 (76%)	47
[a]Three prescreening cases have no pathology confirmation due to missing or bad quality of tumor tissue samples.			

all cohort members was based on the results of direct thyroid measurements, which yielded estimates of the I-131 activities in the thyroid at the time of the measurements and personal interviews (Likhtarev et al., 2006). To calculate the thyroid dose, the variation with time of the I-131 activity was assessed using data from personal interviews (information on residence history, dietary habits, and individual actions taken to reduce doses) and advanced ecological models. Deterministic and stochastic estimates of individual dose were calculated for each subject.

The first estimates of individual thyroid doses (TD-02) for all members of the UkrAm cohort were obtained in 2002 (Likhtarev et al., 2006). The revised thyroid doses (TD-10) (Likhtarov et al., 2014) range from 0.35 mGy to 42 Gy, with 95% of the doses between 1 mGy and 4.2 Gy, an arithmetic mean of 0.65 Gy, and a geometric mean of 0.19 Gy. The most notable improvement of the TD-10 thyroid dosimetry system is a revised assessment of the uncertainties, as shared and unshared error components. Newly developed dose measurement error models make it possible to perform a more realistic risk analysis (Kukush et al., 2011; Little et al., 2014).

FINDINGS AND DISCUSSION

Table 8.3 provides descriptive statistics on the fifth screening cycle. The results of the first four cycles of screening, which have been

Table 8.3 Descriptive Statistics of the Fifth Screening Cycle	
Individual's Status	**Number of Subjects, *n* (%)**
Invited	13,196
Screened	10,073 (76%)
Age at screening, years	26–47
Mean age, years	35
Referred to FNA	554
Completed FNA	447 (81%)
Referred to surgery	108
Completed surgery	82 (76%)
Diagnosis	
Thyroid cancer	47
Thyroid follicular adenoma	33[a]
Thyroid nodule on ultrasound	2,219
[a]Including 10 cases of combined pathology: thyroid cancer and follicular adenoma.	

Table 8.4 Thyroid Cancer Excess Relative Risk (ERR) Estimates in the Framework of UkrAm Study

Reference	Features of Risk Analysis	Time Since Exposure (years)	ERR per Gy	95% CI
Tronko et al. (2006)	Analysis of prevalence cases detected in 1998–2000	12–14	5.25	(1.7; 27.5)
Little et al. (2014)	Analysis of prevalence cases detected in 1998–2000 and contribution of individual doses uncertainties	12–14	4.7–5.8[a]	–
Brenner et al. (2011)	Analysis of incidence cases detected in 2001–08	15–22	1.91	(0.4; 6.3)

[a]ERR variability for three methods of statistical correction of uncertainties in individual doses.

published previously (Tronko et al., 2006; Brenner et al., 2011; Tronko et al., 2012), are summarized in Table 8.4. The analysis of 45 prevalent cases diagnosed at the first screening, indicates an estimated excess relative risk (ERR per Gy) of 5.25 at 12–14 years after exposure (Tronko et al., 2006). Subsequent analysis of 65 incident thyroid cancer cases detected during the second to fourth cycles gives an estimated ERR per Gy of 1.91, indicating that an I-131-related risk was still present 15–22 years after the accident (Brenner et al., 2011). The estimated ERR/Gy for incident thyroid cancer (although lower) was not statistically different from the estimate for prevalent cancer. The persistent excess thyroid cancer risk 15–22 years after I-131 exposure is consistent with the temporal pattern of the risk due to external radiation (Ron et al., 1995), and indicates the importance of continued follow-up of the UkrAm cohort.

During 2012–15, or about 14–17 years after the first examination, the fifth screening cycle was implemented, and 10,116 subjects (76.4% from original cohort size) were examined. Such a relatively high rate of cohort "maintenance" demonstrates the use of effective epidemiological procedures as well as good communication with the cohort members. As mentioned above, the chronology of screening cycles, the number of examined cohort members, and response rate are presented in Table 8.2. The key statistics of the fifth screening are presented in Table 8.3. Descriptive data involve 10,073 cohort members with valid TD-10 dose estimates. Age at examination varied within the range from 26 to 47 years with a mean age of 35 years. According to pathology conclusions, 47 cases of thyroid cancers and 33 cases of follicular adenomas were diagnosed, including 10 cases where more than one type of lesion was present in the same patient, i.e., thyroid cancer and follicular adenoma. In addition, in 2,219 (22.2%) subjects nodular pathology was diagnosed by ultrasound data; about 5.5% of examined subjects were referred to FNA, among them about 81% completed this procedure. According to cytology conclusions, 108 subjects were referred for thyroid surgery; of these, 82 (76%) cohort members were operated on.

Preliminary analysis of the fifth cycle prevalence data indicated that there was a significant I-131 dose−response for thyroid cancer. There was no significant evidence of departure from linearity in dose−response for both malignant and benign thyroid tumors. Assessment of the effect of risk-modifying factors suggests that the risk of development of thyroid neoplasia depends on the age at the time of the accident (being higher for the younger age and decreasing with increasing age), especially in case of follicular adenoma development.

Overall, as of December 2015, in the framework of all cycles of screenings of the UkrAm cohort 179 thyroid cancer cases were diag-nosed (Table 8.2). In addition 14 pre-existing thyroid cancers were operated on and diagnosed in 1990−98 before the initial UkrAm screening had taken place. Among 179 cases of thyroid carcinoma diagnosed for the period 1998−2015, papillary thyroid carcinomas were predominant with 168 cases (93.9%). In addition, nine cases of follicular thyroid carcinoma (5.0%) and two cases of medullary thyroid carcinoma (1.1%) were identified.

The impact of uncertainties in individual doses on risk assessment has been studied by Little et al. (2014). Various methods of statistical correction of ERR estimates (in particular two types of regression cali-bration, Monte Carlo maximum likelihood) show variability in the estimates within the range 8−12%. ERR estimates according to the fifth cycle are consistent with the earlier estimates taking into account the longer time period (26−29 years) after exposure.

The estimated ERR for prevalent thyroid cancer at the first screen-ing in the parallel BelAm cohort ($n = 85$; ERR/Gy = 2.15, 95% CI: 0.81−5.47) (Zablotska et al., 2011) is slightly lower than the corre-sponding value for the UkrAm cohort. However, both values are in general agreement, taking into account the confidence intervals, and are also statistically consistent with the estimated ERR/Gy of 4.7,

(95% CI: 2.5; 7.7) reported in the framework of analytical studies in contaminated regions of Russia (Ivanov et al., 2016). In both the UkrAm and BelAm cohorts, the I-131-related thyroid cancer risk was higher among those exposed at younger than older ages. Other modifying effects (such as residence at the time of the accident, iodine deficiency) were unclear. Pooled analysis of the UkrAm and BelAm thyroid cohorts data will allow us to significantly increase the statistical power in the analysis of the dose−response and risk modification effects, as both studies used a similar methodology.

Presently, the most complete information about the radiation risk of thyroid cancer has been obtained in studies of the external thyroid exposure (Ron et al., 1995; Veiga et al., 2016). The excess thyroid cancer risk associated with childhood exposure in the Japanese atomic bomb survivors has persisted for >50 years after exposure (Furukawa et al., 2013). A significant linear relative risk trend for doses lower than 100 mGy was estimated and radiogenic effects were reported not only for papillary, but also for another types of thyroid cancers (Veiga et al., 2016).

The Chernobyl epidemiological data can provide important information (Ron, 2007; NCRP, 2008; UNSCEAR, 2011) on the magnitude and patterns of the risk from I-131 exposure. Preliminary conclusions on the features of thyroid cancer risk according to the current result of the UkrAm cohort study may be summarized as follows:

- There is a linear "dose−response" relationship between I-131 exposure and risk of thyroid cancer.
- The excess risk remains significant 29 years after I-131 exposure.
- Estimates of relative risk are consistent with other studies of the effects of I-131 exposure and risk estimates from external exposure during childhood.
- A higher risk is assessed for those exposed in the youngest age group.

A further follow-up of cohort members of the Ukrainian−American Thyroid Project is important in order to further our understanding of the dose−effect relationship, the role of risk-modifying factors and to determine the time pattern of the risk in a period of more than 30 years after exposure.

REFERENCES

Astakhova, L.N., Anspaugh, L.R., Beebe, G.W., Bouville, A., Drozdovitch, V.V., Garber, V., et al., 1998. Chernobyl-related thyroid cancer in children of Belarus: a case-control study. Radiat. Res. 150 (3), 349−356.

Brenner, A.V., Tronko, M.D., Hatch, M., Bogdanova, T.I., Oliynik, V.A., Lubin, J.H., et al., 2011. I-131 dose response for incident thyroid cancers in Ukraine related to the Chernobyl accident. Environ. Health Perspect. 119 (7), 933−939. Available from: http://dx.doi.org/10.1289/ehp.1002674.

Bogdanova, T.I., Zurnadzhy, L.Y., Nikiforov, Y.E., Leeman-Neill, R.J., Tronko, M.D., Chanock, S., et al., 2015. Histopathological features of papillary thyroid carcinomas detected during four screening examinations of a Ukrainian-American cohort. Br. J. Cancer 113 (11), 1556−1564. Available from: http://dx.doi.org/10.1038/bjc.2015.372.

Furukawa, K., Preston, D., Funamoto, S., Yonehara, S., Ito, M., Tokuoka, S., et al., 2013. Long-term trend of thyroid cancer risk among Japanese atomicbomb survivors: 60 years after exposure. Int. J. Cancer 132, 1222−1226. Available from: http://dx.doi.org/10.1002/ijc.27749.

Goldman, M., 1997. The Russian radiation legacy: its integrated impact and lessons. Environ. Health Perspect. 105 (Suppl. 6), 1385−1391.

Ivanov, V.K., Kashcheev, V.V., Chekin, S.Y., Maksioutov, M.A., Tumanov, K.A., Meniailo, A.N., et al., 2016. Thyroid cancer: lessons of Chernobyl and projections for Fukushima. Radiat. Risk (Radiatsiya i risk) 24 (2), 8−22 (In Russian).

Jacob, P., Goulko, G., Heidenreich, W.F., Likhtarev, I., Kairo, I., Tronko, N.D., et al., 1998. Thyroid cancer risk to children calculated. Nature 392, 31−32.

Kazakov, V.S., Demidchik, E.P., Astakhova, L.N., 1992. Thyroid cancer after Chernobyl. Nature 359 (6390), 21.

Kukush, A., Shklyar, S., Masiuk, S., Likhtarov, I., Kovgan, L., Bouville, A., 2011. Methods for estimation of radiation risk in epidemiological studies accounting for classical and Berkson errors in doses. Int. J. Biostat. 7 (1), 15. Available from: http://dx.doi.org/10.2202/1557-4679.1281.

Likhtarev, I.A., Sobolev, B.G., Kairo, I.A., Tronko, N.D., Bogdanova, T.I., Oleinic, V.A., et al., 1995a. Thyroid cancer in the Ukraine. Nature 375 (6530), 365.

Likhtarev, I.A., Gulko, G.M., Sobolev, B.G., Kairo, I.A., Prohl, G., Roth, P., et al., 1995b. Evaluation of the I-131 thyroid-monitoring measurements performed in Ukraine during May and June of 1986. Health Phys. 69, 6−15.

Likhtarov, I., Bouville, A., Kovgan, L., Luckyanov, N., Voilleque, P., Chepurny, M., 2006. Questionnaire- and measurement-based individual thyroid doses in Ukraine resulting from the Chornobyl nuclear reactor accident. Radiat. Res. 166, 271−286. Available from: http://dx.doi.org/10.1667/RR3545.1.

Likhtarov, I., Kovgan, L., Masiuk, S., Talerko, M., Chepurny, M., Ivanova, O., et al., 2014. Thyroid cancer study among Ukrainian children exposed to radiation after the Chornobyl accident: improved estimates of the thyroid doses to the cohort members. Health Phys. 106 (3), 370−396. Available from: http://dx.doi.org/10.1097/HP.0b013e31829f3096.

Little, M.P., Kukush, A.G., Masiuk, S.V., Shklyar, S., Carroll, R.J., Lubin, J.H., et al., 2014. Impact of Uncertainties in Exposure Assessment on Estimates of Thyroid Cancer Risk among Ukrainian Children and Adolescents Exposed from the Chernobyl Accident. PLoS One 9 (1), e85723. Available from: http://dx.doi.org/10.1371/. journal.pone.0085723.

Little, M.P., Kwon, D., Zablotska, L.B., Brenner, A.V., Cahoon, E.K., Rozhko, A.V., et al., 2015. Impact of Uncertainties in Exposure Assessment on Thyroid Cancer Risk among Persons in Belarus Exposed as Children or Adolescents Due to the Chernobyl Accident. PLoS One 10 (10), e0139826.

NCRP (National Council on Radiation Protection and Measurements), 2008. Risk to the Thyroid from Ionizing Radiation. NCRP Report No. 159. National Council on Radiation Protection and Measurements, Bethesda, Maryland.

Ron, E., Lubin, J.H., Shore, R., Mabuchi, K., Modan, B., Pottern, L.M., et al., 1995. Thyroid cancer after exposure to external radiation − a pooled analysis of 7 studies. Radiat. Res. 141, 259−277.

Ron, E., 2007. Thyroid cancer incidence among people living in areas contaminated by radiation from the Chernobyl accident. Health. Phys. 93, 502−511. Available from: http://dx.doi.org/10.1097/01.HP.0000279018.93081.29.

Stezhko, V.A., Buglova, E.E., Danilova, L.I., Drozd, V.M., Krysenko, N.A., Lesnikova, N.R., et al., 2004. A cohort study of thyroid cancer and other thyroid diseases after the Chornobyl accident: objectives, design and methods. Radiat. Res. 161 (4), 481−492, http://dx.doi.org/10.1667/3148.

Tronko, M.D., Howe, G.R., Bogdanova, T.I., Bouville, A.C., Epstein, O.V., Brill, A.B., et al., 2006. A cohort study of thyroid cancer and other thyroid diseases after the Chernobyl accident: thyroid cancer in Ukraine detected during first screening. J. Natl. Cancer Inst. 98 (13), 897−903. Available from: http://dx.doi.org/10.1093/jnci/djj244.

Tronko, M., Mabuchi, K., Bogdanova, T., Hatch, M., Likhtarev, I., Bouville, A., et al., 2012. Thyroid cancer in Ukraine after the Chernobyl accident (in the framework of the Ukraine-US Thyroid Project). J. Radiol. Prot. 32 (1), N65−N69. Available from: http://dx.doi.org/10.1088/0952-4746/32/1/N65.

UNSCEAR (United Nations Scientific Committee on the Effects of Atomic Radiation), 2011. Health effects due to radiation from the Chernobyl accident UNSCEAR 2008 Report vol II, Scientific Annex D. United Nations, New York.

Veiga, L., Holmberg, E., Anderson, H., Pottern, L., Sadetzki, S., Adams, J., et al., 2016. Thyroid cancer after childhood exposure to external radiation: an updated pooled analysis of 12 studies. Radiat. Res. 185 (5), 473−484. Available from: http://dx.doi.org/10.1667/RR14213.1.

Zablotska, L.B., Ron, E., Rozhko, A.V., Hatch, M., Polyanskaya, O.N., Brenner, A.V., et al., 2011. Thyroid cancer risk in Belarus among children and adolescents exposed to radioiodine after the Chernobyl accident. Br. J. Cancer 104 (1), 181−187. Available from: http://dx.doi.org/10.1038/sj.bjc.6605967.

CHAPTER 9

Results of the Thyroid Cancer Epidemiological Survey in Russia Following the Chernobyl Accident

Viktor Ivanov[1], Valerii Kashcheev[1], Sergey Chekin[1],
Marat Maksioutov[1], Konstantin Tumanov[1], Alexandr Menyajlo[1],
Oleg Vlasov[1], Elena Kochergina[1], Polina Kashcheeva[1],
Natalia Shchukina[1], Aleksandr Korelo[1], Natalia Seleva[1],
Vsevolod Galkin[1], Andrey Kaprin[2], Vladimir A. Saenko[3]
and Shunichi Yamashita[3]

[1]A. Tsyb MRRC, Obninsk, Russia [2]NMRRC, Obninsk, Russia [3]Nagasaki University, Nagasaki, Japan

INTRODUCTION

The association between radiation and an increase in cancer incidence at high radiation doses has been demonstrated in large-scale epidemiological studies of survivors of the Hiroshima and Nagasaki atomic bombings in 1945. Results of these studies have been used by the UN Scientific Committee on the Effects of Atomic Radiation (UNSCEAR), the International Commission on Radiological Protection (ICRP), and the International Atomic Energy Agency (IAEA) as a basis for establishing international principles of radiation safety.

At the same time, major nuclear power plant accidents, such as those at Three Mile Island, Chernobyl, and Fukushima Daiichi, which have led to radiation exposure of large groups of the local population and employees, have brought to the forefront the issue of estimating possible cancer risks associated with exposure to moderate and low doses of radiation. The development of an evidence-based approach to this issue is critical in identifying high-risk groups, and to develop strategies to provide the necessary and timely medical assistance by healthcare authorities. It also enables using advanced medical technologies to minimize late radiological effects.

Thirty years after the Chernobyl accident, the results of post-Chernobyl epidemiological studies have become even more relevant,

Thyroid Cancer and Nuclear Accidents. DOI: http://dx.doi.org/10.1016/B978-0-12-812768-1.00009-5

since the accumulated knowledge and experience can be used to predict the possible radiological consequences of the Fukushima Daiichi NPP accident in Japan.

The experience gained from the Chernobyl accident has shown that special attention should be given to investigation of thyroid cancer incidence among the population due to the potential exposure to radioiodine released from the reactor. Multiple studies have revealed an increase in thyroid cancer incidence among residents of the areas contaminated by the Chernobyl accident, when compared with baseline national rates in Belarus, Russia, and Ukraine (Ilyin et al., 1990; Kazakov et al., 1992; Tronko et al., 2006; Balonov and Zvonova, 2002; Likhtarov et al., 2006; Jacob et al., 2006a; Cardis et al., 2005). It has also been demonstrated that those who were children at exposure should be regarded as a high-risk group with respect to the development of thyroid cancer following radiation exposure (Likhtarov et al., 2006; Brenner et al., 2011; Zablotska et al., 2011; Jacob et al., 2006b; Walsh et al., 2009; Ivanov et al., 2012; Valentin, 2007).

However, assessment of risks of development of thyroid cancer following low and moderate radiation doses and the prediction of radiation-induced thyroid cancer incidence in subsequent years, given the obvious effects of screening, still remains a significant challenge (Interim Report of Thyroid Ultrasound Examination Initial Screening, 2015; Kashcheev et al., 2015; Ivanov and Kaprin, 2015).

ASSESSMENT OF THE RISK OF THYROID CANCER AND THE EFFECTS OF SCREENING IN THE COHORT DRAWN FROM THE RUSSIAN POPULATION EXPOSED TO RADIATION FOLLOWING THE CHERNOBYL ACCIDENT

This section assesses the screening effect on thyroid cancer incidence among the Russian population due to internal exposure of the thyroid to incorporated radioiodine. These estimates provide a basis for adequate understanding of the results of the childhood thyroid ultrasound examination in Fukushima prefecture.

Fig. 9.1 shows the map of rayon-average thyroid doses received by children and adolescents in the affected rayons of Bryansk, Tula, Kaluga, and Oryol oblasts. As can be seen from the figure, the highest doses were received by children and adolescents in the southwest parts of Bryansk oblast.

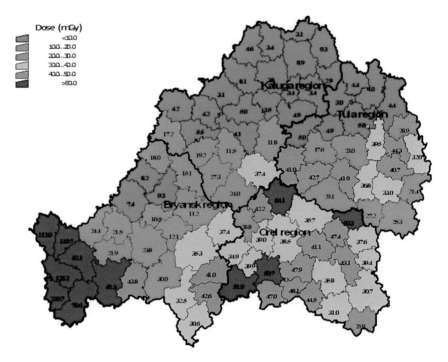

Figure 9.1 Map of mean thyroid doses for children and adolescents (0−17 years) by district (rayon) living in Bryansk, Oryol, Tula, and Kaluga oblasts at the time of the accident.

Fig. 9.2 shows the dose distribution among children and adolescents in seven rayons in the southwest of Bryansk oblast, in which the average dose exceeds 50 mGy.

The methodology used for estimating the screening effect and linear dependence of the increase in thyroid cancer incidence rate on radiation dose is presented in Fig. 9.3.

Based on the cohort regression models (with allowance for sensitivity and specificity) the screening effect and risk of thyroid cancer from radiation exposure were estimated for the studied cohort. The results obtained are shown below. Table 9.1 includes the values of excess relative risks per 1 Gy (ERR/Gy) and screening rates (ES) for children and adolescents at exposure and for adults. As can be seen, significant risk of thyroid cancer induction as a result of radiation exposure has been found only for those who were children and adolescents (0−17 years) at exposure. A higher screening effect (6.74), was observed during the entire follow-up period in the younger age group (0−17 years at exposure) when compared with the rate of 1.5 in those who were adults

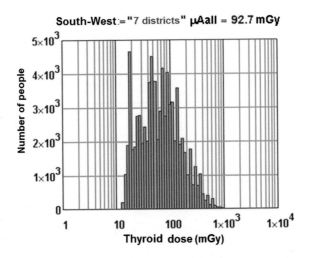

Figure 9.2 Dose distribution among children and adolescents in the districts to the southwest of the Bryansk oblast where the mean thyroid dose is above 50 mGy.

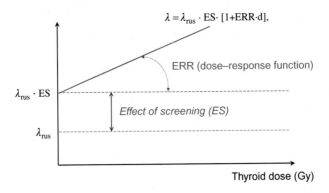

Figure 9.3 Model for assessing the screening effect and linear dependence of the thyroid cancer incidence rate on radiation dose (Kashcheev et al., 2015; Ivanov and Kaprin, 2015).

at exposure. For those who were children and adolescents at exposure the risk of thyroid cancer following radiation exposure has been found to depend significantly on age at exposure and attained age. It should be noted that the screening effect during 1991−95 for children and adolescents was 12.8. A significant ($P<0.001$) twofold decrease in the screening effect, when compared with the first period (1991−95), was observed from 1996.

Fig. 9.4 shows graphically the dependence of the screening effect on calendar time of follow-up of the cohort of children and adolescents at exposure.

Table 9.1 Excess Relative Risks (ERR) and the Effects of Screening (ES) for Thyroid Cancer Incidence in the Cohort From Bryansk, Oryol, Tula, and Kaluga Oblasts During 1991–2013

Follow-up Period: 1991–2013	Children and Adolescents at exposure (0–17 years)	Adults at Exposure (18+ years)
Total number of people	108,166	219,544
Number of cases	316	925
Mean dose for the cohort (mGy)	174	35
Mean dose among the cases (mGy)	190	36
Effect of screening ES, (95% CI), P-value ES1: 1991–95 ES2: 1996–2000 ES3: 2001–05 ES4: 2006–13	 12.8 (8.6; 17.9); $P < 0.001$ 6.6 (4.8; 8.9); $P < 0.001$ 5.8 (4.4; 7.4); $P < 0.001$ 6.8 (5.4; 8.1); $P < 0.001$	 1.3 (0.9; 1.9); $P = 0.11$ 1.2 (1.0; 1.4); $P = 0.04$ 1.9 (1.5; 2.1); $P < 0.001$ 1.6 (1.2; 2.3); $P < 0.001$
ES mean for the period 1991–2013	6.74 (5.6; 7.9); $P < 0.001$	1.5 (1.2; 1.6); $P < 0.001$
ERR/Gy, (95 % CI), P-value	4.73 (2.54; 7.72); $P < 0.001$	-0.60 (-2.93; 1.53); $P = 0.38$
ω, (95% CI), P-value	-2.08 (-3.07; -0.06); $P < 0.001$	-0.12 (-1.17; 1.94); $P > 0.5$
v, (95% CI), P-value	-0.10 (-0.27; 0.01); $P = 0.07$	-0.04 (-0.26; 0.23); $P > 0.5$

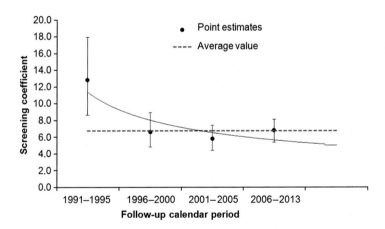

Figure 9.4 Dependence of the effect of screening on the calendar time period of follow-up of the cohort of children and adolescents (0–17 years) at exposure.

The analysis shows that 71 thyroid cancer cases (22.5%) of the detected 316 cases can be attributed to radiation. However, in the age group of 0–4 years at exposure, 52 (60.5%) of 86 thyroid cancer cases detected during the follow-up period from 1991 to 2013 can be attributed to radiation (Table 9.2).

Table 9.2 Fraction of Radiation-Induced Thyroid Cancers Among Children as a Function of Age in 1986			
Age in 1986 (years)	0—4	5—9	10—17
Mean dose (mGy)	326	149	88
Number of detected thyroid cancer cases	86	78	152
Number of radiation-induced thyroid cancers	52	23	4
Fraction of radiation-induced thyroid cancers (%)	60.5	30.0	2.6

REGISTRATION OF THYROID CANCER IN CHILDREN EXPOSED TO RADIATION DUE TO THE FUKUSHIMA DAIICHI NPP ACCIDENT

The fourth volume of the IAEA report into The Fukushima Daiichi Accident (2015) deals with the prediction of possible radiological effects of the accident for the Fukushima Prefecture population. According to the estimates of risk of radiation-induced thyroid cancer, made with the use of ICRP and WHO models and factual Chernobyl data, the magnitude of risk is 0.1% for adults and 1.4% for children against the baseline incidence rate for this disease in Japan (Cancer Statistics in Japan). It was therefore concluded that the likelihood of an increase in thyroid cancer incidence attributable to radiation exposure in Fukushima Prefecture is very low.

In 2011, a large-scale ultrasound thyroid screening program in children and adolescents was initiated in Fukushima Prefecture. During the first round of the diagnostic activity in 2011—13 inclusive a total of 298,577 persons underwent ultrasound examination. As a result, 110 thyroid cancer cases were detected (Interim Report of Thyroid Ultrasound Examination Initial Screening, 2015). Data from the National Radiation Epidemiological Registry (NRER), on thyroid cancer incidence in the population of the most radioactively contaminated oblasts in Russia provided a basis for predicting a number of sporadic (i.e., unrelated to radiation exposure) cases of thyroid cancer in the study cohort of children and adolescents of Fukushima Prefecture, with allowance for the effects of screening.

Using Japanese data from official national statistics (Cancer Statistics in Japan) on operated cases, the average thyroid cancer incidence rate among children and adolescents (0—19 years) in Japan is 2.2 cases per 2 million per year for the respective population. Given the known size of the study cohort, the expected number of spontaneous cancers, with allowance for the screening effect, can be estimated by the following formula:

$$\text{CASES} = \sum_i \text{PYR}_i \lambda_{i(\text{Japan})} \cdot \text{ES} \qquad (9.1)$$

where PYR_i is the follow-up person-years in the i-th group of attained age (0–4, 5–9, 10–14, and 15–19 years) calculated as a product of the study group size by the mean age in the group. $\lambda_{i(\text{Japan})}$ is the thyroid cancer baseline incidence rate in Japan among children and adolescents in the i-th age group, ES is the screening effect in the first period of follow-up of the children and adolescents cohort in four contaminated oblasts of Russia after the Chernobyl accident (ES = 12.8; 95% CI: 8.6; 17.9).

Using the data on the size of the individual age groups from the Interim Report of Thyroid Ultrasound Examination (2015) and thyroid cancer incidence rates averaged over the period from 2000 to 2010 for children and adolescents in Japan (Cancer Statistics in Japan) the number of person-years under follow-up was estimated for the entire cohort. In calculating the number of person-years under follow-up in the group that underwent medical examination in 2012–13, allowance was made for a shift in the screening start date. The total number of person-years of follow-up was 3,018,073.

Table 9.3 shows the results of the predicted sporadic thyroid cancer cases (unrelated to radiation exposure) in the cohort of children and adolescents in Fukushima Prefecture with allowance for the screening

Table 9.3 Prediction of the Number of Sporadic Thyroid Cancer Cases (Unrelated to Radiation) in the Cohort of Children and Adolescents Under Study in Fukushima Prefecture with Allowance for the Effects of Screening and Mean Value of Thyroid Cancer Incidence Rate in Japan (2000–10)

Screening Effect	Number of Children and Adolescents Undertaking Medical Checkup	Number of Detected Thyroid Cancer Cases	Predicted Number of Cases With Allowance for Screening Effect (95% CI)
2011	41,810	15	13.5 (9.0; 18.8)
2012	139,339	56	41.0 (27.6; 57.4)
2013	117,428	39	28.7 (19.3; 40.1)
Total	298,577	110	83.2 (55.9; 116.3)

effect. The table also shows the number of detected thyroid cancer cases based on the results of primary ultrasound screening conducted during the period from October 9, 2011 to March 31, 2014 (Interim Report of Thyroid Ultrasound Examination, 2015). As can be seen from Table 9.3, the predictions and actual data regarding detected thyroid cancer cases are in good agreement.

CONCLUSIONS

The above results have led us to the following conclusions:

1. A significant increase in thyroid cancer incidence rate among the population was detected in the territories of Bryansk, Tula, Kaluga, and Oryol oblasts exposed to higher levels of contamination from radiation after the Chernobyl accident.
2. A significant risk for the development of thyroid cancer following radiation exposure was found for those who were children and adolescents at exposure (0–17 years). It has been found that the radiation risk of thyroid cancer depends on both the age at exposure and attained age for children and adolescents at exposure.
3. A distinct screening effect was identified in the course of thyroid cancer incidence detection (6.74 for children and adolescents 0–17 years at exposure and 1.5 for the group 18 years and older) for the population of most contaminated rayons in Bryansk, Tula, Kaluga, and Oryol oblasts. Estimation of the screening coefficient by follow-up periods has revealed a significant ($P < 0.001$) twofold decrease in the screening effect starting from 1996, as compared with the first period (1991–95).
4. Data from NRER, including estimates of risk of thyroid cancer among children and adolescents exposed to radiation after the Chernobyl accident and the effects of screening were used to predict the likely number of thyroid cancers in Japan after the Fukushima Daiichi NPP accident. The predictions and actual data on detected thyroid cancer cases after the Fukushima accident are in good agreement. These results suggest that the number of thyroid cancer cases detected as a result of thyroid screening in Japan are most likely to reflect the spontaneous incidence of thyroid cancer in that population, rather than an increase related to radiation exposure.

REFERENCES

Balonov, M.I., Zvonova, I.A., 2002. Average Doses of Exposure of the Thyroid Gland of Inhabitants of the Different Age Living in 1986 in Settlements of Bryansk, Tula, Oryol and Kaluga Areas Contaminated by Radionuclides After the Chernobyl Accident: Directory, the Edition Official. Ministry of Health of Russia, Moscow. (*In Russian*).

Brenner, A.V., Tronko, M.D., Hatch, M., Bogdanova, T.I., Oliynik, V.A., Lubin, J.H., et al., 2011. I-131 dose response for incident thyroid cancers in Ukraine related to the Chernobyl accident. Environ. Health Perspect. 119 (7), 933−939.

Cancer Statistics in Japan. Retrieved from <http://www.ncc.go.jp/en/index.html>.

Cardis, E., Kesminiene, A., Ivanov, V., Malakhova, I., Shibata, Y., Khrouch, V., et al., 2005. Risk of thyroid cancer after exposure to ^{131}I in childhood. J. Natl. Cancer Inst. 97 (10), 724−732.

ICRP Publication 103. 2007. Elsevier.

Ilyin, L.A., Balonov, M.I., Buldakov, L.A., Bur'yak, V.N., Gordeev, K.I., Dement'ev, S.I., et al., 1990. Radiocontamination patterns and possible health consequences of the accident at the Chernobyl nuclear power station. J. Radiol. Prot. 10 (1), 3−29.

Interim Report of Thyroid Ultrasound Examination (Initial Screening). 2015. Retrieved from <http://fmu-global.jp/?wpdmdl = 1387>.

Ivanov, V.K., Kaprin, A.D., 2015. Health Effects of Chernobyl: Prediction and Actual Data 30 years After the Accident. GEOS, Moscow, 450 p. (*In Russian*).

Ivanov, V.K., Kashcheev, V.V., Yu, C.S., Maksioutov, M.A., Tumanov, K.A., et al., 2012. Radiation-epidemiological studies of thyroid cancer incidence in Russia after the Chernobyl accident (estimation of radiation risks, 1991−2008 follow-up period). Radiat. Prot. Dosim. 151 (3), 489−499.

Jacob, P., Bogdanova, T.I., Buglova, E., Chepurniy, M., Demidchik, Y., Gavrilin, Y., et al., 2006a. Thyroid cancer risk in areas of Ukraine and Belarus affected by the Chernobyl accident. Radiat. Res. 165 (1), 1−8.

Jacob, P., Bogdanova, T.I., Buglova, E., Chepurniy, M., Demidchik, Y., Gavrilin, Y., et al., 2006b. Thyroid cancer among Ukrainians and Belarusians who were children or adolescents at the time of the Chernobyl accident. J. Radiol. Prot. 26 (1), 51−67.

Kashcheev, V.V., Yu, Chekin, S., Maksiouto, V.M.A., Tumanov, K.A., Korelo, A.M., et al., 2015. Radiation risk and screening effect of thyroid cancer incidence among the population of Bryansk and Orel oblasts of the Russian Federation. Radiat. Risk 24 (1), 8−22 (*In Russian*).

Kazakov, V.S., Demidchik, E.P., Astakhova, L.N., 1992. Thyroid cancer after Chernobyl. Nature 359, 1.

Likhtarov, I., Kovgan, L., Vavilov, S., Chepurny, M., Ron, E., Lubin, J., et al., 2006. Post-Chernobyl thyroid cancers in Ukraine. Report 2: risk analysis. Radiat. Res. 166 (2), 375−386.

The Fukushima Daiichi Accident, 2015. Technical Volume 4/5. Radiological Consequences. IAEA, Vienna, 250 p.

Tronko, M.D., Howe, G.R., Bogdanova, T.I., Bouville, A.C., Epstein, O.V., Brill, A.B., et al., 2006. A cohort study of thyroid cancer and other thyroid diseases after the Chernobyl accident: thyroid cancer in Ukraine detected during first screening. J. Natl. Cancer Inst. 98 (13), 897−903.

Walsh, L., Jacob, P., Kaiser, J.C., 2009. Radiation risk modeling of thyroid cancer with special emphasis on the Chernobyl epidemiological data. Radiat. Res. 172 (4), 509−518.

Zablotska, L.B., Ron, E., Rozhko, A.V., Hatch, M., Polyanskaya, O.N., Brenner, A.V., et al., 2011. Thyroid cancer risk in Belarus among children and adolescents exposed to radioiodine after the Chernobyl accident. Br. J. Cancer 104 (1), 181−187.

CHAPTER 10

Influence of Radiation Exposure and Ultrasound Screening on the Clinical Behavior of Papillary Thyroid Carcinoma in Young Patients

Pavel O. Rumiantsev[1], Vladimir A. Saenko[2] and Ivan I. Dedov[1]

[1]Endocrine Research Centre, Moscow, Russian Federation [2]Nagasaki University, Nagasaki, Japan

The accident at the Chernobyl nuclear power plant occurred over 30 years ago, on April 26, 1986 in the north of Ukraine close to the border with neighboring Belarus and Russia. The most significant health consequence of the accident has been a dramatic increase in the incidence of thyroid cancer among young residents of the regions of the three countries affected by radioactive fallout first observed in the early 1990s. There is now compelling evidence for a causative association between excess thyroid cancer and exposure to ^{131}I from the accident among those exposed in childhood or adolescence. In Russia, four oblasts (the administrative units) were designated as contaminated: Bryansk, Orel, Tula, and Kaluga. According to the National Radiation Epidemiology Registry of Russia, a total of 1241 cases of thyroid cancer have been documented among 327,000 residents during 1991–2013 (Ivanov et al., 2016). These cohort members receive annual comprehensive health checkups, including thyroid ultrasound.

Both radiation exposure and ultrasound screening may increase the incidence of thyroid cancer, although in different ways. Radiation exposure elevates the risk for developing disease through biological processes, while ultrasound screening provides enhanced assessment of otherwise asymptomatic (for most instances) thyroid abnormalities, such as nodules. Here we analyze whether radiation exposure from the Chernobyl accident and ultrasound screening of the thyroid have affected the clinical characteristics of the tumors and evaluate the factors influencing the chance of recurrence of papillary thyroid cancer (PTC) diagnosed in patients from Russia.

Thyroid Cancer and Nuclear Accidents. DOI: http://dx.doi.org/10.1016/B978-0-12-812768-1.00010-1

PATIENTS

We analyzed 717 patients with PTC either exposed to radiation due to the Chernobyl accident or those who lived in other regions of the country, where no radioactive contamination occurred. In 223 cases, PTC was detected in patients of pediatric age (0–17 years at diagnosis) and 494 cases occurred in elder patients (18–38 years old). All the patients were treated from 1983 to 2008 and then followed-up. Inclusion criteria were histologically confirmed PTC and the availability of medical surveillance information. In the pediatric group, the age of the patients varied from 5 to 17 years old (mean 14.3 ± 2.6), and from 18 to 38 years old (mean 27.8 ± 5.4) in young adults. The pediatric group included 75 males and 148 females (M:F ratio 1:1.97). The young adults group included 86 males and 408 females (M:F ratio 1:4.74). The mean follow-up period was 10.0 ± 3.2 and 4.7 ± 3.4 years in the two groups, respectively.

STUDY DESIGN

The aim of this study was to analyze tumor characteristics and recurrence rates in patients with radiation-related (internal exposure to radioiodine after Chernobyl) and sporadic PTC, and to compare those between the group of PTCs "actively" detected by ultrasound screening with those identified without screening.

Patients were divided into two age groups (pediatric and young adults) and each group into two subgroups in order to evaluate the impact of both factors (radiation exposure and screening effect) in the different age groups separately. The criteria of radiation-induced PTC (RI-PTC) were living at the moment of the Chernobyl disaster in contaminated territories and reconstructed individual thyroid dose >50 mGy (51–3170 mGy, range), while those of sporadic PTC (SP-PTC) were living in noncontaminated regions of Russia, or had radiation dose to the thyroid <5 mGy or were born after the accident. Two other subgroups were formed to compare patients who did not participate in any ultrasound screening program with those who underwent annual screening (designated NS-PTC and S-PTC, respectively). The pediatric group was abbreviated as PD (PD-RI-PTC and PD-SP-PTC) and the young adults group as YA (YA-RI-PTC and YA-SP-PTC). Tumor staging was according to the seventh edition of UICC pTNM classification (Sobin et al., 2010). Statistical analysis was performed with SPSS ver. 22.0 software (IBM SPSS Statistics, USA).

RESULTS

In the pediatric group (PD-group), age at diagnosis was not statically different between the subgroups under comparison (i.e., radiation-induced/sporadic and screened/nonscreened), whereas in the young adults group (YA-group) there was a significant difference between radiation-induced (RI) and sporadic (SP) subgroups (25.5 vs. 28.6 years old, $P < 0.0001$). Sex ratio was significantly shifted toward males in the PD-S-PTC as compared to the PD-NS-PTC group (M:F 1:1.26 vs. 1:2.60, $P = 0.011$). Mean tumor size was significantly smaller in PD-S-PTC than in PD-NS-PTC subgroups (13.9 vs. 16.9 mm, $P = 0.017$) but not between PD-RI-PTC and PD-SP-PTC (14.3 vs. 16.1, $P = 0.18$). Tumor stage was not significantly different between PD-PTC subgroups.

Tumor size in the YA-PTC group was significantly smaller in the YA-RI-PTC than in the YA-SP-PTC subgroup (11.4 vs. 14.0, $P = 0.01$) as well as in the YA-S-PTC than in the YA-NS-PTC subgroups (11.7 vs. 14.8, $P = 0.0006$). This was paralleled by the higher prevalence of microcarcinoma (<1 cm, pT1a) in both YA-RI-PTC and YA-S-PTC vs. YA-SP-PTC and YA-NS-PTC subgroups (57.6% vs. 46.6%, $P = 0.04$; and 57.3% vs. 42.3%, $P = 0.006$, respectively). More advanced tumor stages (pT2 and pT3) were more frequent in the YA-RI-PTC vs. YA-SP-PTC subgroups (5.6% vs. 14.1%, $P = 0.01$; and 4.0% vs. 10.8%, $P = 0.02$, respectively). Nodal disease (N1 category) and distant metastases (M1 category) were less frequent in the YA-S-PTC than in the YA-NS-PTC subgroup (48.1% vs. 62.0%, $P = 0.0021$; and 0% vs. 2.7%, $P = 0.016$, respectively). It is worth noting that PTC with lymph node spread beyond the central compartment (N1b) was about twofold more frequent in the YA-NS-PTC than in the YA-S-PTC subgroup (26.9% vs. 16.5%, $P < 0.0001$).

Histologically, in the pediatric age group, the classical variant of PTC was significantly less frequent in the PD-RI-PTC vs. the PD-SP-PTC group (55.1% vs. 70.8%, $P = 0.032$). The follicular variant was marginally more frequent in RI-PTC vs. SP-PTC and S-PTC vs. NS-PTC subgroups (36.2% vs. 22.7%, $P = 0.049$; and 34.0% vs. 21.4%,

$P = 0.047$, respectively). Of note, diffuse chronic autoimmune thyroiditis as a background process in the thyroid was less frequently seen in the PD-RI-PTC and PD-S-PTC vs. the PD-SP-PTC and PD-NS-PTC subgroups (5.8% vs. 16.2%, $P = 0.033$; 7.2% vs. 17.5%, $P = 0.028$, respectively). In young adult patients, the classical variant of PTC was less frequent in the YA-S-PTC subgroup than in the YA-NS-PTC subgroup (62.4% vs. 77.3%, $P = 0.0004$). In contrast, the follicular variant was more common in the YA-S-PTC vs. the YS-NS-PTC subgroup (29.9% vs. 16.5%, $P = 0.0006$). Similarly to the pediatric age group, diffuse chronic autoimmune thyroiditis was less frequent in the YA-S-PT subgroup than in YA-NS-PTC (13.7% vs. 21.5%, $P = 0.026$).

The clinical treatment of the patient was comparable between PD-PTC subgroups. In contrast, in the YA-PTC subgroups subtotal thyroidectomy was performed less frequently in the YA-RI-PTC vs. the YA-SP-PTC subgroup (0.8% vs. 6.0%, $P = 0.014$). Central neck dissection was done more frequently in the YA-RI-PTC than in the YA-SP-PTC subgroup (83.2% vs. 74.0%, $P = 0.039$). This difference can be explained by the fact that most patients in the RI-PTC subgroup were treated in the federal medical center while most patients with SP-PTC were operated in local hospitals. Lateral neck dissections were performed more frequently in YA-NS-PTC patients than in the YA-S-PTC subgroup (26.9% vs. 14.1%, $P = 0.0005$). Likely due to the higher proportion of more advanced disease (M1, N1b) in the YA-NS-PTC than in the YA-S-PTC subgroup, patients of the former subgroup received radioiodine treatment more frequently (41.5% vs. 30.8%, $P = 0.015$).

Tumor recurrence rate (8 years, mean follow-up period) was significantly lower in the PD-S-PTC group as compared to the PD-NS-PTC group (18.6% vs. 31.7%, $P = 0.031$; OR = 0.49, 95% CI: 0.26–0.92). Cox regression analysis revealed that the chance of recurrence was significantly lower in PD-S-PTC vs. PD-NS-PTC (HR = 0.86, 95% CI: 0.76–0.97, $P = 0.016$). Similar results of disease-free survival (mean follow-up period, 4.7 years) were obtained in the YA-PTC subgroup analysis. There was no difference between the RI and SP subgroups. However, there was statistically significant difference between the YA-S-PTC and YA-NS-PTC subgroups (7.7% vs. 20.4%, $P < 0.0001$; OR = 0.33, 95% CI: 0.18–0.57). Cox proportional hazard model confirmed a significantly lower chance of recurrence among screened vs.

nonscreened young adult patients (HR $= 0.84$, 95% CI: 0.74–0.94, $P = 0.003$).

DISCUSSION

Both radiation exposure and ultrasound screening of the thyroid are the factors increasing thyroid cancer incidence. We conducted a comparative analysis of demographic, clinico-morphological parameters and of recurrence-free survival of PTC patients of various age groups (pediatric and young adults at the moment of diagnosis) in order to assess the influence of radiation exposure and ultrasound screening effects separately.

Most cases in the pediatric group (0–18 years old at the moment of the accident) were diagnosed after 1993–1994. At that time, two diagnostic centers were established in the most contaminated in Russia Bryansk region in Klintsy city and in Bryansk city. The majority of patients with nodules revealed by ultrasound and confirmed as cancerous or suspicious for cancer by fine-needle aspiration biopsy were directed for treatment to the Medical Radiological Research Center, Obninsk.

Radiation and screening factors both shifted the F:M ratio toward the male gender in the pediatric group. Mean tumor size was significantly decreased in the screened vs. nonscreened pediatric PTC group. In the YA-PTC-group not only mean tumor size but also T1 tumor stage were significantly more frequent in radiation-induced and screened subgroups. Lateral lymph node involvement (N1b) was more common in the nonscreened than in the screened subgroup among young adults. Moreover, among young adults screened by ultrasound there were no cases with distant metastases, which is in contrast with the nonscreened group. This indicates that patients with tumors detected by ultrasound screening could benefit from early diagnosis and either early intervention or close monitoring (Yuen et al., 2011).

The analysis of disease-free survival did not reveal unfavorable influence of radiation exposure either in the pediatric or young adult age groups, which is in line with our earlier study (Rumyantsev et al., 2011). However, ultrasound screening seems to decrease the chance of recurrence in these groups of young patients (Tables 10.1 and 10.2).

Table 10.1 Comparison of Demographic, Clinico-morphological, Treatment, and Recurrence-Free Survival Data in the Pediatric Group of PTC Patients

Parameters	PD-RI-PTC Subgroup, abs.	PD-SP-PTC Subgroup, abs.	OR (95% CI)	P	PD-S-PTC Subgroup, abs.	PD-NS-PTC Subgroup, abs.	OR (95% CI)	P
Number of Patients	69	154	NA	NA	97	126	NA	NA
M:F	28:41	47:107	1.56 (0.86−2.81)	0.17	43:54	35:91	2.07 (1.18−3.62)	0.011
Age, years	14.22 ± 2.81	14.40 ± 2.53	NA	0.65	14.23 ± 2.71	14.44 ± 2.53	NA	0.59
Size, mm	14.30 ± 8.83	16.08 ± 9.66	NA	0.18	13.90 ± 7.50	16.89 ± 10.47	NA	0.014
pT0	0	1 (0.6%)	NS	1.00	0	1 (0.8%)	NS	1.00
pT1a	27 (39.1%)	52 (33.8%)	NS	0.45	38 (39.2%)	41 (32.5%)	NS	0.33
pT1b	24 (34.8%)	56 (36.4%)	NS	0.88	37 (38.1%)	43 (34.1%)	NS	0.57
pT2	7 (10.1%)	27 (17.5%)	NS	0.23	11 (11.3%)	23 (18.3%)	NS	0.19
pT3	10 (14.5%)	17 (11.0%)	NS	0.51	9 (9.3%)	18 (14.3%)	NS	0.30
pT4	1 (1.4%)	1 (0.6%)	NS	0.52	2 (2.1%)	0	NS	0.19
N0	25 (36.2%)	57 (37.0%)	NS	1.00	37 (38.1%)	45 (35.7%)	NS	0.78
N1a	21 (30.4%)	44 (28.6%)	NS	0.87	31 (32.0%)	34 (27.0%)	NS	0.46
N1b	23 (33.3%)	53 (34.4%)	NS	1.00	29 (29.9%)	47 (37.3%)	NS	0.26
M1	8 (11.6%)	18 (11.7%)	NS	1.00	10 (10.3%)	16 (12.7%)	NS	0.68
Txm (tumor multifocality)	20 (29.0%)	54 (35.1%)	NS	0.44	27 (27.8%)	47 (37.3%)	NS	0.15
Encapsulated tumors	11 (15.9%)	22 (14.3%)	NS	0.84	15 (15.5%)	18 (14.3%)	NS	0.85
Classical variant	38 (55.1%)	109 (70.8%)	0.51 (0.28−0.91)	0.03	59 (60.8%)	88 (69.8%)	NS	0.20
Follicular variant	25 (36.2%)	35 (22.7%)	1.93 (1.04−3.59)	0.05	33 (34.0%)	27 (21.4%)	1.89 (1.04−3.44)	0.047

Diffuse-sclerosing variant	3 (4.3%)	4 (2.6%)	NS	0.68	2 (2.1%)	5 (4.0%)	NS	0.70
Solid variant	3 (4.3%)	5 (3.2%)	NS	0.70	3 (3.1%)	5 (4.0%)	NS	0.70
Other histological variants	0	1 (1.4%)	NS	1.0	0	1 (0.8%)		1.00
Diffuse chronic thyroiditis	4 (5.8%)	25 (16.2%)	**0.32** (0.11–0.95)	**0.03**	7 (7.2%)	22 (17.5%)	**0.37** (0.15–0.90)	**0.028**
Focal thyroiditis	1 (1.4%)	11 (7.1%)	NS	0.11	6 (6.2%)	6 (4.8%)	NS	0.77
Graves' disease	0	2 (1.3%)	NS	1.0	1 (1.0%)	1 (0.8%)	NS	1.00
Thyroid lobe resection	0	6 (3.9%)	NS	0.18	1 (1.0%)	5 (4.0%)	NS	0.24
Hemithyroidectomy	27 (39.1%)	67 (43.5%)	NS	0.56	40 (41.2%)	54 (42.9%)	NS	0.89
Subtotal thyroidectomy	3 (4.3%)	6 (3.9%)	NS	1.0	4 (4.1%)	5 (4.0%)	NS	1.00
Total thyroidectomy	39 (56.5%)	75 (48.7%)	NS	0.31	52 (53.6%)	62 (49.2%)	NS	0.59
Central lymph node dissection	56 (81.2%)	105 (68.2%)	NS	0.05	76 (78.4%)	85 (67.5%)	NS	0.10
Lateral lymph node dissection	24 (34.8%)	58 (37.7%)	NS	0.76	32 (33.0%)	50 (39.7%)	NS	0.33
Radioiodine treatment	41 (59.4%)	71 (46.1%)	NS	0.08	51 (52.6%)	61 (48.4%)	NS	0.59
Follow-up period, years	9.9 ± 3.3	7.2 ± 5.4	NA	–	9.2 ± 4.20	7.8 ± 5.4	NA	–
Tumor recurrence, frequency	13 (18.8%)	45 (29.2%)	NS	0.14	18 (18.6%)	40 (31.7%)	**OR 0.49** (0.26–0.92)	**0.031**
Disease-free survival							**HR 0.86** (0.76–0.97)	**0.016**

Values in bold emphasize the differences between samples that are statistically significant.

Table 10.2 Comparison of demographic, clinico-morphological, treatment, and recurrence-free survival data in young adults with PTC

Parameters	YA-RI-PTC Subgroup. abs.	YA-SP-PTC Subgroup. abs.	OR (95% CI)	P	YA-S-PTC Subgroup. abs.	YA-NS-PTC Subgroup. abs.	OR (95% CI)	P
Number of Patients	125	369	NA	NA	234	260	NA	NA
M:F	24:101	62:307	NS	0.59	41:193	45:215	NS	1.00
Age, years	25.5 ± 5.2	28.6 ± 5.1	NA	<0.0001	27.7 ± 5.3	28.0 ± 5.5	NA	0.54
Size, mm	11.4 ± 8.4	14.0 ± 10.7	NA	0.0058	11.7 ± 8.9	14.8 ± 11.1	NA	0.0006
pT0	1 (0.8%)	1 (0.3%)	NS	0.44	1 (0.4%)	1 (0.4%)	NS	1.00
pT1a	72 (57.6%)	172 (46.6%)	1.56 (1.03–2.34)	0.039	134 (57.3%)	110 (42.3%)	1.83 (1.28–2.61)	0.0012
pT1b	39 (31.2%)	102 (27.6%)	NS	0.49	63 (26.9%)	78 (30.0%)	NS	0.49
pT2	7 (5.6%)	52 (14.1%)	0.36 (0.16–0.82)	0.01	23 (9.8%)	36 (13.8%)	NS	0.21
pT3	5 (4.0%)	40 (10.8%)	0.34 (0.13–0.89)	0.02	13 (5.6%)	32 (12.3%)	0.42 (0.21–0.82)	0.01
pT4	1 (0.8%)	2 (0.5%)	NS	1.00	0	3 (1.2%)	NS	0.25
N0	64 (51.2%)	206 (55.8%)	NS	0.41	145 (62.0%)	125 (48.1%)	1.76 (1.23–2.52)	0.0021
N1a	39 (31.2%)	86 (23.3%)	NS	0.095	60 (25.6%)	65 (25.0%)	NS	0.92
N1b	22 (17.6%)	77 (20.9%)	NS	0.52	29 (12.4%)	70 (26.9%)	0.38 (0.24–0.62)	<0.0001
M1	2 (1.6%)	5 (1.4%)	NS	1.0	0	7 (2.7%)	0.07 (0.004–1.27)	0.016
Txm (tumor multifocality)	37 (29.6%)	119 (32.2%)	NS	0.66	65 (27.8%)	91 (35.0%)	NS	0.1
Encapsulated tumors	38 (30.4%)	118 (32.0%)	NS	0.82	82 (35.0%)	74 (28.5%)	NS	0.12

Classical variant	82 (65.6%)	265 (71.8%)	NS	0.21	146 (62.4%)	201 (77.3%)	0.49 (0.33–0.72)	**0.0004**
Follicular variant	33 (26.4%)	80 (21.7%)	NS	0.32	70 (29.9%)	43 (16.5%)	**2.15** (1.4–3.31)	**0.0006**
Diffuse-sclerosing variant	5 (4.0%)	6 (1.6%)	NS	0.16	4 (1.7%)	7 (2.7%)	NS	0.55
Solid variant	4 (3.2%)	10 (2.7%)	NS	0.76	7 (3.0%)	7 (2.7%)	NS	1.00
Other histological variants	1 (0.8%)	8 (2.2%)	NS	0.40	7 (3.0%)	2 (0.8%)	NS	0.092
Diffuse chronic thyroiditis	16 (12.8%)	72 (19.5%)	NS	0.1	32 (13.7%)	56 (21.5%)	**0.58** (0.36–0.93)	**0.026**
Focal thyroiditis	12 (9.6%)	32 (8.7%)	NS	0.72	22 (9.4%)	22 (8.5%)	NS	0.75
Graves' disease	1 (0.8%)	3 (0.8%)	NS	1.00	0	4 (1.5%)	NS	0.13
Thyroid lobe resection	1 (0.8%)	3 (0.8%)	NS	1.00	1 (0.4%)	3 (1.2%)	NS	0.63
Isthmusectomy	0	6 (1.6%)	NS	0.36	4 (1.7%)	2 (0.8%)	NS	0.43
Hemithyroidectomy	64 (51.2%)	151 (40.9%)	NS	0.048	116 (49.6%)	99 (38.1%)	**1.6** (1.12–2.29)	**0.011**
Subtotal thyroidectomy	1 (0.8%)	22 (6.0%)	**0.13** (0.02–0.95)	**0.014**	7 (3.0%)	16 (6.2%)	NS	0.13
Total thyroidectomy	59 (47.2%)	187 (50.7%)	NS	0.54	106 (45.3%)	140 (53.8%)	NS	0.059
Central lymph node dissection	104 (83.2%)	273 (74.0%)	**1.74** (1.03–2.94)	**0.039**	185 (79.1%)	192 (73.8%)	NS	0.2
Lateral lymph node dissection	23 (18.4%)	80 (21.7%)	NS	0.52	33 (14.1%)	70 (26.9%)	**0.45** (0.28–0.71)	**0.0005**
Radioiodine treatment	40 (32.0%)	140 (37.9%)	NS	0.24	72 (30.8%)	108 (41.5%)	**0.63** (0.43–0.91)	**0.015**

(*Continued*)

Table 10.2 (Continued)

Parameters	YA-RI-PTC Subgroup. abs.	OR (95% CI)	P	YA-SP-PTC Subgroup. abs.	OR (95% CI)	P	YA-S-PTC Subgroup. abs.	YA-NS-PTC Subgroup. abs.	OR (95% CI)	P
Number of Patients	**125**	NA	NA	**369**	NA	NA	**234**	**260**	NA	NA
Follow-up period, years	4.9 ± 3.0	NS	0.36	4.6 ± 3.5	NS	0.36	4.7 ± 3.2	4.7 ± 3.5	NS	1.00
Tumor recurrence, frequency	17 (13.6%)	NS	0.88	54 (14.6%)	NS	0.88	18 (7.7%)	53 (20.4%)	**OR 0.33** (0.18–0.57)	**< 0.0001**
Disease-free survival									**HR 0.84** (0.74–0.94)	**0.003**

Values in bold emphasize the differences between samples that are statistically significant.

CONCLUSIONS

Based on these observations, we conclude that radiation exposure does not influence the chance of recurrence. Ultrasound screening has a moderate favorable effect on not only earlier tumor detection but also on disease-free survival in both pediatric and young adult age groups of patients with PTC. Further follow-up of patients is necessary to clarify the influence of radiation and screening on the chance of recurrence and overall survival at longer time points.

REFERENCES

Ivanov, V.K., Kashcheev, V.V., Yu, C.S., Maksyutov, M.A., Tumanov, K.A., et al., 2016. Thyroid cancer: lessons of Chernobyl and projections for Fukushima. Radiat. Risk 25 (2), 5–19 (Russian).

Rumyantsev, P.O., Saenko, V.A., Ilyin, A.A., Stepanenko, V.F., Rumyantseva, U.V., Abrosimov, A.Y., et al., 2011. Radiation exposure does not significantly contribute to the risk of recurrence of Chernobyl thyroid cancer. J. Clin. Endocrinol. Metab. 96 (2), 385–393. Available from: http://dx.doi.org/10.1210/jc.2010-1634.

Sobin, L.H., Gospodarowicz, M.K., Wittekind, C., International Union against Cancer, 2010. TNM Classification of Malignant Tumours, seventh ed. Wiley-Blackwell, Chichester, West Sussex, UK; Hoboken, NJ.

Yuen, A.P., Ho, A.C., Wong, B.Y., 2011. Ultrasonographic screening for occult thyroid cancer. Head Neck 33 (4), 453–457. Available from: http://dx.doi.org/10.1002/hed.21462.

CHAPTER 11

Results of Treatment in Children and Adolescents With Differentiated Thyroid Carcinoma Not Exposed and Exposed to Radiation From the Chernobyl Accident

Christoph Reiners[1], Johannes Biko[1], Yuri E. Demidchik[2,4] and Valentina M. Drozd[2,3]

[1]University of Würzburg, Würzburg, Germany [2]Belarusian Medical Academy of Postgraduate Education, Minsk, Belarus [3]The International Fund "Help for Patients with Radiation Induced Thyroid Cancer "Arnica", Minsk, Belarus [4]Republican Centre for Thyroid Tumors, Minsk, Belarus

INTRODUCTION

It is generally accepted that children are vulnerable to induction of thyroid cancer by external or internal exposure to radiation (Veiga et al., 2016). The 2011 Fukushima Nuclear Power Plant accident raised public health concerns about an increased incidence of differentiated thyroid carcinoma (DTC) in the exposed pediatric population and about the prognosis of affected individuals (Normile, 2016). The latter concerns might be addressed by comparing experience with thyroid cancer in children and adolescents following the 1986 Chernobyl Nuclear Power Plant accident to the clinical course of thyroid cancer in controls of similar age not exposed to Chernobyl radiation.

Contrary to the situation following the Fukushima accident in 2011, iodine-131 contamination of milk and lack of appropriate counter-measures after the Chernobyl accident led to high thyroid doses in the general public, particularly in children (Balonov, 2007; Bennett et al., 2006; Cardis et al., 2006; Sources and Effects of Ionizing Radiation, 2008) Consequently, approximately 5 years later, DTC incidence began to substantially increase among those exposed as juveniles. In children under age 14 years in 1986, 5127 new DTC cases were reported from 1991 to 2005 for Belarus, Ukraine, and the four most affected Russian Federation regions (Balonov, 2007; Bennett et al., 2006; Cardis et al., 2006; Demidchik et al., 2007; Ron, 2007; Sources and Effects of

Thyroid Cancer and Nuclear Accidents. DOI: http://dx.doi.org/10.1016/B978-0-12-812768-1.00011-3

Ionizing Radiation, 2008). By 1995, DTC incidence in children under age 10 years increased to 40 per 1,000,000 per year (Cardis et al., 2006; Demidchik et al., 2007), compared to, e.g., 1–5 per 1,000,000 per year in the United States (Surveillance, Epidemiology, and End Results SEER Program, 2010).

On the other hand, recently a considerable number of thyroid findings have been described in children and adolescents in the context of thyroid screening as part of the Fukushima Health Survey (including thyroid cancer) even if the radiation doses in these subjects have been very low (Suzuki et al., 2016). Up to now, this effect most probably can be explained by screening bias and not by exposure to radiation from the Fukushima reactor emergency (Normile, 2016).

Our main objective here is to analyze the disease status, response to therapy, and mortality in Chernobyl cases (Demidchik et al., 2006; Hebestreit et al., 2011; Reiners et al., 2008, 2013; Reiners, 2009) to a historic control group from the literature summarizing therapy results from different studies in children and adolescents not exposed to Chernobyl fallout. Parts of this comparison already have been published elsewhere (Reiners et al., 2013).

MATERIALS AND METHODS
Historic Controls
The historic control group from the literature includes 1976 cases from 15 studies published between 1997 and 2015 (Chow et al., 2004; Dottorini et al., 1997; Grigsby et al., 2002; Handkiewicz-Junak et al., 2000, 2007; Hay et al., 2010; La Quaglia et al., 2000; Mihailovic et al., 2014; Newman et al., 1998; Popovtzer et al., 2006; Reiners et al., 2013; Segal et al., 1998; Vaisman et al., 2011; Vassilopoulo-Sellin et al., 1998; Verburg et al., 2015; Wada et al., 2009) (Table 11.1), which were compiled after a systematic literature search for treatment and follow-up in children with differentiated thyroid cancer not exposed to Chernobyl radiation before the onset of the disease.

Patients Exposed to Chernobyl radiation
The group exposed to Chernobyl fallout involves in total 1305 children and adolescents from three studies reported between 2000 and 2013 (Demidchik et al., 2006; Reiners et al., 2013; Rybakov et al., 2000) (Table 11.1). The most recent follow-up study about Chernobyl

Table 11.1 Presentation, Treatment, and Outcome of Differentiated Thyroid Cancer in Children and Adolescents (Studies With More Than 50 Patients Published After 1990)

Author, Reference	Year of Publication	Patients	Mean Age (Years)	Mean Follow-Up (Years)	Papillary Histology (%)	pTNM Stage T4 (%)	pTNM Stage N1 (%)	pTNM Stage M1 (%)	Total Resection (%)	Therapy LN Dissection	Therapy I-131 Therapy	Therapy LT4 Medication	Remission Rate (%)	All-Cause Mortality Rate (%)
Dottorini	1997	85	15	9	85	31	60	19	59	n.a.	89	Most	74	0
Vassilopoulo	1998	112	15	25	92	38	63	28	73	62	Most	Most	93	12
Segal	1998	61	16	n.a.	79	26	49	6	83	59	100	100	94	4
Newman	1998	329	15	11	90	32	74	25	54	56	43	n.a.	67	1
La Quaglia selection M1	2000	327	15	11	90	48	90	100	66	51	100	100	69	1
Jarzab	2000	109	14	5	71	n.a.	59	16	74	100	100	100	61	0
Grigsby	2002	56	16	11	95	54	60	13	92	95	82	100	61	2
Chow	2004	60	17	14	82	23	45	15	82	87	60	100	91	3
Popovtzer	2006	75	16	n.a.	83	n.a.	60	6	89	100	89	100	87	3
Handkiewicz	2007	235	15	7	82	8	40	17	73	67	74	100	86	1
Wada	2009	120	16	12	89	13	62	8	51	89	15	91	77	0
Hay	2010	215	16	29	100	18	78	6	89	86	35	n.a.	68	10
Vaisman	2011	65	14	13	69	40	62	29	100	50	100	n.a.	67	0
Mihailovic	2014	51	17	10	94	24	67	14	94	67	90	100	90	6
Verburg	2015	76	16	12	87	9	50	22	91	50	91	100	67	0
Rybakov	2000	330	ca.12	ca.5	94	55	62	15	84	57	75	100	93	2
Demidchik	2006	741	12	10	95	16	69	18	58	82	63	100	72	1
Reiners	2012	234	12	11	99	64	97	43	85	78	100	100	63	1

I-131, iodine-131; LN, lymph node; LT4, levothyroxine; n.a., not available. Shaded rows denote Chernobyl-induced disease; studies summarized in unshaded rows involved patients with "sporadic" disease.

patients was published in 2013 by ourselves, including 234 selected patients with advanced disease (Demidchik et al., 2006). Exposure to radiation from the Chernobyl accident took place in infancy or young childhood (median age 1.6 years). After surgery in Belarus the patients received radioiodine therapy (RIT) in Germany; they were followed-up in Belarus and Germany.

For comparison, the weighted medians of time measured in years and percentages respectively are presented in the following text.

RESULTS

Historic Controls

For interpretation of the data, the study of La Quaglia et al. (2000) (Table 11.1) will not be taken into account because this was a selected study in children and adolescents with severely advanced, metastatic disease which is not typical for this age group (see below). Therefore, finally the study cohort consists of 14 studies with 1649 patients.

The median age at diagnosis of this cohort (Table 11.1) is 16 years and median follow-up time 11 years. A high percentage of patients (88%) show papillary histology. At presentation 28% of the cohort are diagnosed with local invasion (stage pT4), 61% with neck lymph node involvement (N1), and 17% with distant metastases (M1).

With respect to treatment protocols 73% of the patients receive total thyroidectomy and 69% lymph node dissection, followed by RIT in 64% and thyroid hormone substitution in close to 100%.

Concerning therapy outcome and follow-up reported in the 14 studies from the literature, the median rates for remission are 75% and 3% for all-cause mortality. It should be mentioned in this context, that two studies by Vassilopoulo-Sellin et al. (1998) and Hay et al. (2010) showed higher all-cause mortalities of 12% and 10%, respectively, during very long follow-ups of 25 and 29 years, respectively. It is self-explaining, however, that during such a long follow-up "natural" mortality exceeds tumor-related mortality.

Patients Exposed to Chernobyl Radiation

The search resulted in three follow-up studies of 1305 children and adolescents who developed thyroid cancer after exposure to Chernobyl radiation

(Table 11.1). The median age at diagnosis of 12 years is remarkably younger than in the control cohort. The patients are followed-up for a median time of 10 years. A higher percentage of exposed patients (96%) as compared to controls (88%) show papillary histology.

With respect to the stage of the disease, our publication from 2013 (Reiners et al., 2013; last row of Table 11.1) has to be discussed separately, since these patients represent a highly selective group with advanced stages of disease.

At presentation, out of the DTC 1071 patients of the two nonselective studies by Rybakov et al. (2000) and Demidchik et al. (2006), 28% were diagnosed with local invasion (stage pT4), 67% with neck lymph node involvement (N1), and 17% with distant metastases (M1). These signs of aggressiveness seem to be no more prominent in the exposed group when compared to controls with 28%, 61%, and 17% respectively.

The percentage of patients receiving total thyroidectomy (66%) is somewhat lower than in the control group (73%), whereas lymph nodes are dissected (74%) slightly more frequently than in controls with 69%. Radioiodine is given after surgery in 67% of the exposed patients with similar frequency to controls (64%). All patients in the exposed group received thyroid hormone substitution.

Concerning therapy outcome and follow-up reported in the studies about Chernobyl patients, the median rates for remission are 78% and for all-cause mortality 2%, which again is very similar to the results in pediatric patients not exposed to Chernobyl radiation with 75% and 3%, respectively.

In the selected cohort of 234 patients with advanced DTC after Chernobyl (Reiners et al., 2013; Table 11.1 last row), the median age at diagnosis of 12 years again is remarkably young; the latency time since the reactor accident is 11 years. Median follow-up time in this group is 11 years. Virtually all thyroid cancers (99%) showed papillary histology. Due to the selection of patients with advanced disease, 64% of the cohort showed local invasion (stage pT4) at presentation and 97% neck lymph node involvement. At final staging following whole-body scintigraphy after I-131 therapy, 43% of the patients selected because of aggressive disease showed iodine-avid distant metastases, involving the lungs in all cases, plus the bone in two cases and the brain in one.

Not surprisingly, the rate of remission with 63% in these advanced stages is lower than in less aggressive cancers of the exposed (78%) and nonexposed groups (75%). However, all-cause mortality of 1% is as low as in less aggressive cancers of the exposed (1%) and even lower than in the nonexposed group (3%).

DISCUSSION

Historic Controls

According to studies published during the last 25 years, the life-time prognosis of differentiated thyroid cancer (quoad vitam) in children and adolescents is generally very good with all-cause mortality rates as low as 0%–3%, irrespective of radiation exposure as the possible cause of this disease (Table 11.1). Concerning remission, the picture is not so homogeneous with remission rates varying between 65% and 95% reported in the more recent studies from the last 25 years (Table 11.1).

With respect to possible influence factors however, Handkiewicz-Junak et al. (2007) in a study on 235 patients from Poland showed that thyroidectomy and RIT are independent significant predictors of success (Farahati et al., 2000). Similarly, Chow et al. (2004) demonstrated that locoregional recurrences after 20 years in pediatric patients treated with radioiodine with a rate of 20% are significantly less frequent than with 56% in a comparable group without RIT. F. Verburg from our group provided evidence that female gender, lower tumor stage, and successful thyroid ablation by radioiodine are predictors of remission (Verburg et al., 2015).

Interestingly, when comparing the historic controls (Table 11.1) with respect to the application of RIT ($<65\%$ vs $>65\%$ of the patients receiving such treatment), the median remission rates are 71% and 84% in favor of "more prevalent RIT." This difference is highly significant ($P < .001$, Chi-square test).

Patients Exposed to Chernobyl Radiation

Generally, the percentage of patients with papillary histology close to 100% is higher in "Chernobyl children" with thyroid cancer than in the control group. This phenomenon was thought to be caused by radiation exposure; however, prevailing papillary histology is related to young age of thyroid cancer patients (Farahati et al., 2000) and could also be explained by the age difference between the Chernobyl group (median age 12 years) and the control group (median age 16 years).

This comparative cohort study involves some of the highest-risk juveniles with Chernobyl radiation-induced DTC (Williams, 2008). Due to the selection criteria (Reiners et al., 2013) for iodine-131 treatment in Germany, this cohort had frequent local invasion (64% pT4 disease) and distant metastasis (43%) and nearly universal nodal involvement (97%). In the early years after the reactor accident, due to a lack of surgical equipment and requisite facilities and medication, e.g., radioiodine and thyroid hormones, in Belarus, a considerable proportion of patients had suboptimal treatment before RIT in Germany: incomplete surgery, no or only low-activity postsurgical RIT, intermittent or nonsuppressive thyroid hormone therapy, and even percutaneous irradiation or chemotherapy with ineffective drugs. Many early patients (Demidchik et al., 2006) had advanced disease with distant metastases and high initial Tg concentration. Additionally, the interval between tumor excision and the first RIT in Germany—more than half a year on average—was longer than is generally recommended (Francis et al., 2015; Franzius et al., 2007; Higashi et al., 2011; Luster et al., 2007).

Nonetheless, our key finding is that despite the unfavorable prognostic characteristics of our patients and their often suboptimal initial care, final treatment results after application of state-of-the-art RIT protocols were very good. All 229 patients evaluable for outcome responded to the combination of surgical resection, iodine-131 therapy, and suppressive levothyroxine. Today, after a median follow-up of over 12 years, 63% are in complete remission, 30% in nearly complete remission, and 5% in partial remission. We observed only two recurrencies, both local, which responded well to additional 131-therapy so avoiding progression.

To identify variables influencing the course of the disease, we performed multivariate analyses on the outcome groups "complete remission," "nearly complete remission," and "partial remission" and on the extent of RIT. The probabilities for nearly complete remission or even complete response increased with the time span between exposure and diagnosis (i.e., the clinical latency period), an earlier disease stage, and a lower initial Tg level as surrogate of T-stage, defined as a postoperative determination performed immediately before the first RIT in Germany ($P < .01$, Kruskal–Wallis analysis).

These results seem to compare favorably with those published after similar follow-up durations for large cohorts with less advanced sporadic juvenile thyroid cancer. In these reports, all-cause mortality of 0%–3% resembled that in our more severely ill sample, but remission rates mostly were higher, ranging from 65% to 95% (Table 11.1). However, taking into account the advanced tumor stages of our patients with 64% local aggressiveness, 97% lymph node, and 43% distant metastases, the remission rate of 63% may be considered satisfying.

Other than two individuals expiring of apparently thyroid cancer-unrelated causes, the only death in our cohort was a patient succumbing to pulmonary fibrosis as an RIT side effect (Hebestreit et al., 2011; Reiners et al., 2013). Pulmonary fibrosis has previously been reported in thyroid cancer patients who had pulmonary metastases and received therapeutic radioiodine. Since the younger patients in our intensively surveilled subgroup were at an increased risk to develop pulmonary fibrosis with iodine-131 treatment, and young age might be a risk factor for the development of fibrosis with lung irradiation, it is likely that the radiation from iodine-131 accumulating in pulmonary metastases induced fibrotic changes (Pawelczak et al., 2010). The case of fatal pulmonary fibrosis underlines the need for awareness of this side effect after RIT in children with disseminated pulmonary metastases (Biko et al., 2011). In addition, continuous monitoring of children and adolescents after treatment with high doses of RIT is necessary because of a treatment-related possible increased risk for leukemia and solid tumors, such as breast cancer (Kumagai et al., 2007).

To conclude, this survey underlines the recommendations of the American Thyroid Association Management Guidelines for Children with Thyroid Nodules and Differentiated Thyroid Cancer published in 2015 (Francis et al., 2015) which recommend to consider radioiodine ablation seriously in children with locally invasive or extensive lymph node involvement and state that radioiodine is mandatory in surgically noncurable locally advanced tumors as well as in incompletely removed lymph nodes and distant metastases with I-131 uptake.

Interpretation

The Chernobyl reactor accident raised fears of a "radiation-induced pediatric thyroid cancer epidemic" causing high mortality; similar concerns emerged following the Fukushima accident. However, our long-term observational study in a large group of Belarusian juveniles with advanced radiation-induced DTC suggests that even when such disease is advanced and initially suboptimally treated, outcomes are generally favorable after appropriate RIT. With respect to the Fukushima incident, due to timely countermeasures (sheltering, evacuation, and a ban on potentially contaminated food and milk), the risk of radiation-induced DTC in children is much lower than it was after Chernobyl (Nagataki, 2016) and—if there were any increased pediatric thyroid cancer incidence related to exposure by the Fukushima accident at all—it is very likely that due to early DTC diagnosis by screening, advanced cases would be avoided.

REFERENCES

Balonov, M., 2007. Third annual Warren K Sinclair keynote address: retrospective analysis of impacts of the Chernobyl accident. Health Phys. 93, 383–409.

Bennett, B., Repacholi, M., Carr, Z., 2006. Health Effects of the Chernobyl Accident and Special Health Care Programmes. Report of the UN Chernobyl Forum Expert Group "Health.". World Health Organization, Geneva.

Biko, J., Reiners, C., Kreissl, M.C., Verburg, F.A., Demidchik, Y., Drozd, V., 2011. Favourable course of disease after incomplete remission on (131)I therapy in children with pulmonary metastases of papillary thyroid carcinoma: 10 years follow-up. Eur. J. Nucl. Med. Mol. Imag. 38, 651–655.

Cardis, E., Howe, G., Ron, E., Bebeshko, V., Bogdanova, T., Bouville, A., et al., 2006. Cancer consequences of the Chernobyl accident: 20 years on. J. Radiol. Prot. 26, 127–140.

Chow, S.M., Law, S.C., Mendenhall, W.M., Au, S.K., Yau, S., Mang, O., et al., 2004. Differentiated thyroid carcinoma in childhood and adolescence-clinical course and role of radioiodine. Pediatr. Blood Cancer 42, 176–183.

Demidchik, Y.E., Demidchik, E.P., Reiners, C., Biko, J., Mine, M., Saenko, V.A., et al., 2006. Comprehensive clinical assessment of 740 cases of surgically treated thyroid cancer in children of Belarus. Ann. Surg. 243, 525–532.

Demidchik, Y.E., Saenko, V.A., Yamashita, S., 2007. Childhood thyroid cancer in Belarus, Russia, and Ukraine after Chernobyl and at present. Arq. Bras. Endocrinol. Metab. 51, 748–762.

Dottorini, M.E., Vignati, A., Mazzucchelli, L., Lomuscio, G., Colombo, L., 1997. Differentiated thyroid carcinoma in children and adolescents: a 37-year experience in 85 patients. J. Nucl. Med. 38, 669–675.

Farahati, J., Demidchik, E.P., Biko, J., Reiners, C., 2000. Inverse association between age at the time of radiation exposure and extent of disease in cases of radiation-induced childhood thyroid carcinoma in Belarus. Cancer 88, 1470–1476.

Francis, G.L., Waguespack, S.G., Bauer, A.J., Angelos, P., Benvenga, S., Cerutti, J.M., et al., 2015. Management guidelines for children with thyroid nodules and differentiated thyroid cancer. Thyroid 25, 716–759.

Franzius, C., Dietlein, M., Biermann, M., Frühwald, M., Linden, T., Bucsky, P., et al., 2007. Procedure guideline for radioiodine therapy and I-131 iodine whole-body scintigraphy in pediatric patients with differentiated thyroid cancer. Nuklearmedizin 46, 224–231.

Grigsby, P.W., Gal-or, A., Michalski, J.M., Doherty, G.M., 2002. Childhood and adolescent thyroid carcinoma. Cancer 95, 724–729.

Handkiewicz-Junak, D., Wloch, J., Roskosz, J., Krajewska, J., Kropinska, A., Pomorski, L., et al., 2000. Multivariate analysis of prognostic factors for differentiated thyroid carcinoma in children. Eur. J. Nucl. Med. 27, 833–841.

Handkiewicz-Junak, D., Wloch, J., Roskosz, J., Krajewska, J., Kropinska, A., Pomorski, L., et al., 2007. Total thyroidectomy and adjuvant radioiodine treatment independently decrease locoregional recurrence risk in childhood and adolescent differentiated thyroid cancer. J. Nucl. Med. 48, 879–888.

Hay, I.D., Gonzalez-Losada, T., Reinalda, M.S., Honetschlager, J.A., Richards, M.L., Thompson, G.B., 2010. Long-term outcome in 215 children and adolescents with papillary thyroid cancer treated during 1940 through 2008. World J. Surg. 34, 1192–1202.

Hebestreit, H., Biko, J., Drozd, V., Demidchik, Y., Burkhardt, A., Trusen, A., et al., 2011. Pulmonary fibrosis in youth with juvenile thyroid cancer after Chernobyl. Eur. J. Nucl. Med. Mol. Imag. 38, 1683–1690.

Higashi, T., Nishii, R., Yamada, S., Nakamoto, Y., Ishizu, K., Kawase, S., et al., 2011. Delayed initial radioactive iodine therapy resulted in poor survival in patients with metastatic differentiated thyroid carcinoma: a retrospective statistical analysis of 198 cases. J. Nucl. Med. 52, 683–689.

Kumagai, A., Reiners, C., Drozd, V., Yamashita, S., 2007. Childhood thyroid cancers and radioactive iodine therapy: necessity of precautious radiation health risk management. Endocr. J. 54, 839–847.

La Quaglia, M.P., Black, T., Holcomb 3rd, G.W., Sklar, C., Azizkhan, R.G., Haase, G.M., et al., 2000. Differentiated thyroid cancer: clinical characteristics, treatment and outcome in patients under 21 years of age who present with distant metastases. A report from the Surgical Discipline Committee of the Children's Cancer Group. J. Pediatr. Surg. 35, 955–959.

Luster, M., Lassmann, M., Freudenberg, L.S., Reiners, C., 2007. Thyroid cancer in childhood: management strategy, including dosimetry and long-term results. Hormones (Athens) 6, 269–278.

Mihailovic, J., Nikoletic, K., Srbovan, D., 2014. Recurrent disease in juvenile differentiated thyroid carcinoma: prognostic factors, treatments, and outcomes. J. Nucl. Med. 55, 710–717.

Nagataki, S., 2016. Minimizing the Health Effects of the Nuclear Accident in Fukushima on Thyroids. Eur. Thyroid. 5, 219–223.

Newman, K.D., Black, T., Heller, G., Azizkhan, R.G., Holcomb 3rd, G.W., Sklar, C., et al., 1998. Differentiated thyroid cancer: determinants of disease progression in patients <21 years of age at diagnosis: a report from the Surgical Discipline Committee of the Children's Cancer Group. Ann. Surg. 227, 533–541.

Normile, D., 2016. Epidemic of fear. Science 351, 1022–1023.

Pawelczak, M., David, R., Franklin, B., Kessler, M., Lam, L., Shah, B., 2010. Outcomes of children and adolescents with well-differentiated thyroid carcinoma and pulmonary metastases following I-131 treatment: a systematic review. Thyroid 20, 1095–1101.

Popovtzer, A., Shpitzer, T., Bahar, G., Feinmesser, R., Segal, K., 2006. Thyroid cancer in children: management and outcome experience of a referral center. Otolaryngol Head Neck Surg 135, 581–584.

Reiners, C., 2009. Radioactivity and thyroid cancer. Hormones (Athens) 8, 185–191.

Reiners, C., Biko, J., Haenscheid, H., Hebestreit, H., Kirinjuk, S., Baranowski, O., et al., 2013. Twenty-five years after Chernobyl: outcome of radioiodine treatment in children and adolescents with very high-risk radiation-induced differentiated thyroid carcinoma. J. Clin. Endocrinol. Metab. 98, 3039–3048.

Reiners, C., Demidchik, Y.E., Drozd, V.M., Biko, J., 2008. Thyroid cancer in infants and adolescents after Chernobyl. Minerva Endocrinologica 33, 381–395.

Ron, E., 2007. Thyroid cancer incidence among people living in areas contaminated by radiation from the Chernobyl accident. Health Phys. 93, 502–511.

Rybakov, S.J., Komissarenko, I.V., Tronko, N.D., Kvachenyuk, A.N., Bogdanova, T.I., Kovalenko, A.E., et al., 2000. Thyroid cancer in children of Ukraine after the Chernobyl accident. World J. Surg. 24, 1446–1449.

Segal, K., Shvero, J., Stern, Y., Mechlis, S., Feinmesser, R., 1998. Surgery of thyroid cancer in children and adolescents. Head Neck 20, 293–297.

Sources and Effects of Ionizing Radiation. United Nations Scientific Committee on the Effects of Atomic Radiation 2001 UNSCEAR 2008 report to the general assembly with scientific annexes, Volume II Annex D: Health effects due to radiation from the Chernobyl accident. New York: United Nations.

Surveillance, Epidemiology, and End Results (SEER) Program (www.seer.cancer.gov) Research Data (1992-2007), National Cancer Institute, DCCPS, Surveillance Research Program, Cancer Statistics Branch, released April 2010, based on the November 2009 submission.

Suzuki, S., Suzuki, S., Fukushima, T., Midorikawa, S., Shimura, H., Matsuzuka, T., et al., 2016. Comprehensive survey results of childhood thyroid ultrasound examinations in fukushima in the first four years after the fukushima daiichi nuclear power plant accident. Thyroid 26, 843–851.

Vaisman, F., Bulzico, D.A., Pessoa, C.H., Bordallo, M.A., Mendonça, U.B., Dias, F.L., et al., 2011. Prognostic factors of a good response to initial therapy in children and adolescents with differentiated thyroid cancer. Cinics (São Paulo) 66, 281–286.

Vassilopoulo-Sellin, R., Goepfert, H., Raney, B., Schultz, P.N., 1998. Differentiated thyroid cancer in children and adolescents: clinical outcome and mortality after long-term follow-up. Head Neck 20, 549–555.

Veiga, L.H., Holmberg, E., Anderson, H., Pottern, L., Sadetzki, S., Adams, M.J., et al., 2016. Thyroid cancer after childhood exposure to external radiation: an updated pooled analysis of 12 studies. Radiat Res 185, 473–484.

Verburg, F.A., Mäder, U., Luster, M., Hänscheid, H., Reiners, C., 2015. Determinants of successful ablation and complete remission after total thyroidectomy and ^{131}I therapy of paediatric differentiated thyroid cancer. Eur. J. Nucl. Med. Mol. Imag. 4, 1390–1398.

Wada, N., Sugino, K., Mimura, T., Nagahama, M., Kitagawa, W., Shibuya, H., et al., 2009. Treatment strategy of papillary thyroid carcinoma in children and adolescents: clinical significance of the initial nodal manifestation. Ann. Surg. Oncol. 16, 3442–3449.

Williams, D., 2008. Twenty years experience with post-Chernobyl thyroid cancer. Best. Pract. Res. Clin. Endocrinol. Metabol. 22, 1061–1073.

FURTHER READING

Reiners, C., 2003. Radioiodine therapy in patients with pulmonary metastases of thyroid cancer: when to treat, when not to treat? Eur. J. Nucl. Med. Mol. Imag. 30, 939–942.

CHAPTER 12

Somatic Genomics of Childhood Thyroid Cancer

Gerry Thomas
Imperial College London, London, United Kingdom

Thyroid cancer comprises about 3.8% of all new malignancies and is most commonly diagnosed between 45 and 54 years of age, but its incidence is rising in a number of developed countries, including the United States (https://seer.cancer.gov/statfacts/html/thyro.html). Thyroid cancer in those who are under 14 years of age at diagnosis is even rarer, of the order of 0.5−1 per million per year, but varies across the world (Muir et al., 1987). However, within 5 years following the accident at the Chernobyl nuclear power plant on April 26, 1986, there was an unprecedented increase in the rate of pediatric thyroid cancer, mainly papillary thyroid cancer (PTC), in northern Ukraine and southern Belarus (Kazakov et al., 1992; Baverstock et al., 1992). The reason for this was undoubtedly exposure to radioiodine in fallout. The explosion and fire in the graphite core of the reactor had led to the release of more than 10^{19} Bequerels (Bq) of radioisotopes including 1.8×10^{18} Bq of 131-iodine, 2.5×10^{18} Bq 133-iodine, and 1.1×10^{18} Bq 132- Tellurium, which decays to 132-iodine (UNSCEAR, 2000). Iodine is concentrated and bound in the human thyroid from about 3 months of intrauterine age; for this reason, exposure to the thyroid from ^{131}I is 1000−2000 times the average body dose (Braverman and Untiger, 1991). ^{131}I has a short physical half-life, which results in quick elimination from the environment. Patients who were born more than 9 months after the accident were therefore not exposed to radioiodine either in utero or as young children. Many of the children in the exposed areas of Belarus, Ukraine, and Russia received thyroid doses in excess of 1 Gy (UNSCEAR, 2008). The thyroid is known to be a particularly radiosensitive tissue. Studies following the atomic bombs in Japan in the 1940s have shown that those exposed under the age of 10, carried a higher risk of developing thyroid cancer until they were

Thyroid Cancer and Nuclear Accidents. DOI: http://dx.doi.org/10.1016/B978-0-12-812768-1.00012-5

aged 40 (Thompson et al., 1994). The BEIR VII model of the risk of radiation-induced thyroid cancer (Committee to Assess Health Risks from Exposure to Low Levels of Ionizing Radiation, 2006) based on studies of groups of children exposed to external sources of radiation (Ron et al., 1995) predicts a lifetime excess relative risk (ERR) of around 10 per Gy for exposure in early childhood, falling to an ERR of about 2 per Gy at age 20 at exposure. The reason for this differential risk is not known, but is believed to result from a combination of factors, including the mitotic activity of the tissue at exposure.

The Chernobyl accident provided the opportunity not only to better understand the reasons for the relatively higher risk from radiation exposure in the young, but also the genomics of early-onset thyroid cancer. It is clear that in the absence of radiation exposure, pediatric thyroid cancer and adult-onset thyroid cancer are clinically different entities as evidenced by the production of two distinct treatment guidelines by the American Thyroid Association (Haugen et al., 2016; Francis et al., 2015). Since the clinical behavior of cancers is known to be related to their molecular biology, it might therefore be postulated that young-onset thyroid cancer might be genomically distinct from adult-onset disease. Many researchers have speculated that tumors produced as a result of radiation exposure would show a specific molecular profile. For other cancer types such as breast cancer (McGuire et al., 2015) and acute myeloid leukemia (Grimwade et al., 2016) there are clear differences in molecular phenotype associated with the age of the patient at diagnosis. Grimwade et al. (2016) state that cytogenetic analyses of large cohorts of AML patients have shown that translocations/inversions underlie disease pathogenesis in $\sim 50\%$ and 30% of AML arising in children and younger adults, respectively, whereas only a minority of AMLs presenting in older adults carry balanced rearrangements. The Thyroid Cancer Genome Atlas consortium published a large review of PTC that included a small number of young patients, aged under 30 at diagnosis. Their analysis showed that translocations were more frequently found in the youngest patients, and point mutation was more common in older patients. They commented that the frequency of translocations was lower than in PTCs from patients exposed to radiation from the Chernobyl accident. However, their findings were based on a small number of patients ($n = 44$) under the age of 30 at diagnosis of which only 10 were aged under 20 at diagnosis (Cancer Genome Atlas Network, 2014).

Obtaining large numbers of human biological samples is key to dissecting out the molecular mechanisms involved in oncogenesis. Due to the rarity of thyroid cancer in young people, and therefore the difficulty in obtaining sufficient biological material, prior to the Chernobyl accident, there had been little focus on the differences between the genomics of thyroid cancer in patients of different ages. The Chernobyl Tissue Bank (CTB: www.chernobyltissuebank.com) was established in 1998 to provide access to a large number of pathologically reviewed and quality-assured biological samples with information on radiation doses. The collection of samples is prospective and also includes samples from patients who were born after the Chernobyl accident and resident in the same areas of Ukraine and Russia. Because ^{131}I has a short physical half-life, the levels of radiation attributable to radioiodine released from the accident decay in the environment after 3 months. Therefore those children born after January 1, 1987 are not considered to have been exposed to radioiodine from the accident. This group provides the "control" population used in studies to identify whether the genomic pattern observed in these tumors is more likely to be linked to radiation exposure or to age of the patient at diagnosis.

SOMATIC GENOMICS OF YOUNG-ONSET PAPILLARY THYROID CANCER

This chapter will focus only on the somatic genomics of childhood PTC. There have been few studies of statistically appropriate size that have focused on the role of germline genetics on thyroid cancer in the young. A review of these studies was included in a chapter published elsewhere (Schoetz et al., 2014).

The majority of thyroid cancers that have arisen post-Chernobyl are PTCs. The detailed pathology of these tumors has been reviewed before (LiVolsi et al., 2011). In brief, there is a clear association between the morphology of PTC and the age of the patient, with PTCs showing a predominantly solid morphology more common in young children, and the frequency of the classical type of PTC increasing with increasing age. Morphologically, post-Chernobyl PTCs are not dissimilar when compared with those from an age-matched series from England and Wales, but are strikingly different when compared to those from an age-matched series from Japan (Williams et al., 2004).

This suggests that the morphology of these tumors may owe more to dietary iodine (Williams et al., 2008) and/or underlying germline genetics than to exposure to radiation per se. Research thus far suggests that alterations in the MAP kinase signaling pathway are the major drivers of growth in PTC, both in adult- and young-onset tumors. Mutations in the *BRAF* oncogene, or translocations involving the *RET* oncogene predominate; both activate this pathway.

STUDIES ON MAP KINASE PATHWAY ACTIVATION

Initial studies (Nikiforov et al., 1997; Fugazzola et al., 1995, Klugbauer et al., 1995) reported a higher than expected frequency of *RET* rearrangement in post-Chernobyl thyroid cancer, suggesting some *RET* rearrangements might be regarded as a marker for radiation exposure. More recent papers however, have suggested that there is no link between radiation exposure and *RET* rearrangements (Fenton et al., 2000; Williams et al., 1996; Powell et al., 2005). Instead, the high prevalence of one particular type of rearrangement of the *RET* gene (*RET/PTC3*) in post-Chernobyl PTC may reflect the association between the solid morphological subtype with *RET/PTC3* rearrangement and the age of the patient at diagnosis, rather than the etiology of the tumor (Nikiforov et al., 1997; Powell et al., 2005).

There have been few statistically valid studies of *RET* rearrangement in non-Chernobyl-associated pediatric thyroid cancers (Nikiforov et al., 1997; Fenton et al., 2000; Williams et al., 1996), making substantiation of the association of *RET* rearrangements with age at diagnosis difficult. The correlation between molecular biology and pathology is not absolute: in all of the series published so far, a substantial proportion (30%–50%) of the papillary cancers do not harbor a *RET* rearrangement. A variety of different techniques have been used to assess the frequency of *RET* rearrangements and, although this may explain the variation in frequency observed among studies (Zhu et al., 2006), there still remains a large proportion of papillary thyroid carcinomas for which alternative molecular pathways needed to be identified. In addition, it has also been suggested that *RET* rearrangements are not found in all cells in post-Chernobyl papillary carcinomas, and that cells harboring the rearrangement may be clustered (Unger et al., 2004). The degree of clustering appears to be related to the latency of the tumors, with tumors of shorter latency giving a more homogeneous profile than those of longer latency (Unger et al., 2006). This suggests either a polyclonal origin of these tumors or that *RET* rearrangement is a later event in thyroid papillary carcinogenesis than had previously been thought.

The most frequently mutated gene in adult thyroid cancer is the *BRAF* oncogene, but the frequency varies from 36% to 69% (Cohen et al., 2009; Kimura et al., 2003), including one study on Ukrainian tumors (Powell et al., 2005). *BRAF* mutation in post-Chernobyl cases (aged under 18 at operation) is much lower, less than 10% (Powell et al., 2005), and does not appear to be significantly different from that observed in sporadic childhood thyroid papillary carcinoma (Kumagai et al., 2004; Lima et al., 2004). A small number of childhood PTCs have also been shown to harbor a translocation of the *BRAF* oncogene (Ciampi et al., 2005).

One study, which included the cohort of patients who were born after December 1, 1987, suggests that *RET* rearrangement is indeed associated with young age at diagnosis and the solid phenotype of papillary thyroid carcinoma (Powell et al., 2005). Taken together with the BRAF results on post-Chernobyl PTCs, these results have led us to conclude that (1) *RET* rearrangement and *BRAF* mutation are not related to exposure to radiation, but show a strong association with age of the patient at operation; (2) *RET* rearrangement and *BRAF* mutation are mutually exclusive; and (3) *RAS*, *RET*, and *BRAF* oncogenes, although they all activate the MAPK pathway, are associated with tumors of different pathological phenotypes. One possible explanation is that activation via *RET* is more likely to provide a growth advantage to the tumor in the child's thyroid, whereas *BRAF* is more likely to produce a growth advantage in the adult thyroid. These results suggest that crosstalk with pathways other than MAPK may be an important factor in thyroid tumor growth at different ages and that using molecular techniques that have become available in the last decade to study multiple alterations in a single tumor will provide more insight.

Although *RET/PTC* and *BRAF* alterations are the commonest oncogene alterations seen in PTC, rearrangements and mutations of other genes that signal through the MAPK pathway are also observed, but at a much lower frequency. *NTRK1* encodes the high-affinity nerve growth factor receptor, and is occasionally rearranged in PTC. The *NTRK1* rearrangement is only present in about 11% of sporadic PTCs

(Beimfohr et al., 1999) and is rare (3.3%) in post-Chernobyl thyroid tumors (Rabes et al., 2000; Alberti et al., 2003; Pierotti and Greco, 2006). The most recent studies have shown that translocations involving the *NTRK3* gene and *ETV6* may also have a role to play in thyroid carcinogenesis in the young (Ricarte-Filho et al., 2013; Leeman-Neill et al., 2014), although whether this is related to radiation exposure is unclear.

Other types of thyroid cancer are known to involve much different oncogenes, such as the *RAS* oncogene (Lemoine et al., 1989) in follicular carcinoma or *TP53* (encodes p53) in anaplastic carcinoma (Ito et al., 1992). Mutations of the thyroid-stimulating hormone receptor gene (*TSHR*) occur in follicular carcinoma and benign thyroid tumors (Parma et al., 1995; Russo et al., 1995) A large study by Santoro et al. (2000) showed that alteration in none of these genes was present in the post-Chernobyl PTC cohort. Other studies could also not demonstrate correlation of TSH receptor or p53 mutations in thyroid carcinogenesis after radiation exposure (Hillebrandt et al., 1997; Smida et al., 1997; Suchy et al., 1998; Nikiforov et al., 1996). *RAS* mutations are not commonly found in sporadic PTC except for the follicular variant of PTC, although they are identified in benign follicular thyroid tumors, and detection in radiation-induced childhood PTC is similarly rare (Kumagai et al., 2004; Suchy et al., 1998; Fenton et al., 1999).

DNA COPY NUMBER ALTERATIONS

DNA copy number studies on CTB material have suggested that there are distinct chromosomal copy number alterations that correlate with *RET* rearrangement status and that these vary among PTCs diagnosed in adults and those diagnosed in childhood and adolescence. Stein et al. (2010) used tumor and matching normal tissue of 10 Ukrainian patients with post-Chernobyl PTC to examine copy number changes and gene expression. The latency for these tumor patients was 13−14 years, and age at exposure varied from 3 months to 18 years, whereas age at operation was from 14 to 31. Several amplifications on chromosome 22 were detected in all 10 samples. Chromosomes 1 and 12q showed amplifications with high frequency, but less frequent amplifications on 5p, 9q, 16p, and 21q were also detected. Deletions were identified in chromosomes 21q and 14q, and two tumors showed deletions on other chromosomes. In general, deletions are less common in PTC than amplifications, irrespective of radiation exposure. Hieber et al. (2011) examined chromosomal aberrations and *RET/PTC* rearrangements in a cohort of 23 patients from Ukraine who developed PTC after the Chernobyl accident. The median age of the patients at operation was 21. The study revealed chromosomal aberrations in 14 of the cases, most frequently on chromosome 7, 10, 11, 21, and 22. No control group of sporadic PTC was included in this study. Although radiation is thought to generate an increased amount of deletions, translocations, and inversions due to chromosomal damage, these studies show no direct evidence that the number of chromosomal aberrations in radiation-induced PTC is higher than in sporadic PTC. This may be partially due to the design of the studies as confounders such as age at operation, ethnic origin, and histology of the tumor play a major role in the molecular phenotype of tumors and the cohorts studied often lack matched controls. One further study, conducted with an appropriate control group, and using BAC array, has indicated that radiation could potentially be associated with gain of part of chromosome 7 (Hess et al., 2011), although this was only identified in about a third of the cases exposed to radiation. This finding has yet to be validated in other studies that include a nonexposed group of patients of similar age.

GENE EXPRESSION

Studies using CTB material to look at RNA profiles have yielded conflicting results, with some groups suggesting that RNA profiles from radiation-associated cancers are different from age-matched controls (Ricarte-Filho et al., 2013; Handkiewicz-Junak et al., 2016), whilst others have suggested that a radiation fingerprint can be observed in the normal tissue rather than the tumor (Dom et al., 2012). Through collaboration with the US-supported Ukraine–American cohort, a series of papers have been produced suggesting a linkage between molecular biological features and dose, although these papers lacked a nonirradiated control group (Abend et al., 2012, 2013; Leeman-Neill et al., 2013; Selmansberger et al., 2015a). The most recently published results have suggested that the *CLIP2* gene should be considered as a marker for tumors of a radiation etiology (Selmansberger et al., 2015b; Kaiser et al., 2016). However, these studies require further independent validation. Studies are currently underway in partnership with the Cancer Genome Atlas consortium which will result in detailed whole-genome profiling of 500 PTCs—450 from CTB patients exposed to radioiodine in fallout and 50 who were not exposed—and should result in validation (or otherwise) of the results summarized above. Preliminary results are expected in 2017.

SUMMARY

The increase in PTCs in young children and adolescents following the Chernobyl accident provided the opportunity to develop a better understanding of the genomics of this type of thyroid cancer and to investigate whether the molecular biology was driven by etiology or by the age of the patient. In the early studies, assumptions were made about the attribution of the molecular phenotype to radiation. Over the last decade, the rapid developments in genomics, and improved access to large, well-annotated collections of human biological samples of cancers, has increased our understanding of how age affects the molecular phenotype of cancers in general. As a result, many molecular changes that were suggested previously to be biomarkers of radiation in post-Chernobyl PTCs may be in the process of being reclassified as being related more to the age of the patient at diagnosis. This may help us to provide biological reasons why the clinical behavior, and therefore the treatment of PTC in children, should be different from that in the adult. The advances in genomics should result in more tailored treatment and better outcomes for patients, as well as a fascinating biological insight into how the physiology of the individual affects cancer development.

REFERENCES

Abend, M., Pfeiffer, R.M., Ruf, C., Hatch, M., Bogdanova, T.I., Tronko, M.D., et al., 2012. Iodine-131 dose dependent gene expression in thyroid cancers and corresponding normal tissues following the Chernobyl accident. PLoS One 7 (7), e39103.

Abend, M., Pfeiffer, R.M., Ruf, C., Hatch, M., Bogdanova, T.I., Tronko, M.D., et al., 2013. Iodine-131 dose-dependent gene expression: alterations in both normal and tumour thyroid tissues of post-Chernobyl thyroid cancers. Br. J. Cancer 109 (8), 2286–2294.

Alberti, L., Carniti, C., Miranda, C., Roccato, E., Pierotti, M.A., 2003. RET and NTRK1 proto-oncogenes in human diseases. J. Cell Physiol. 195 (2), 168–186.

Baverstock, K., Egloff, B., Pinchera, A., Williams, D., 1992. Thyroid cancer after Chernobyl. Nature 359, 21–22.

Beimfohr, C., Klugbauer, S., Demidchik, E.P., Lengfelder, E., Rabes, H.M., 1999. NTRK1 re-arrangement in papillary thyroid carcinomas of children after the Chernobyl reactor accident. Int. J. Cancer 80 (6), 842–847.

Braverman, L.E., Untiger, R.D. (Eds.), 1991. The Thyroid, a Fundamental and Clinical Text. 6th edn JD Lippincott, Philadelphia.

Cancer Genome Atlas Research Network, 2014. Integrated genomic characterization of papillary thyroid carcinoma. Cell 159 (3), 676−690.

Ciampi, R., Knauf, J.A., Kerler, R., Gandhi, M., Zhu, Z., Nikiforova, M.N., et al., 2005. Oncogenic *AKAP9-BRAF* fusion is a novel mechanism of MAPK pathway activation in thyroid cancer. J. Clin. Invest. 115 (1), 94−101.

Cohen, Y., Xing, M., Mambo, E., Zhongmin, G., Wu, G., Trink, B., et al., 2009. BRAF mutation in papillary thyroid carcinoma. J. Natl. Cancer Inst. 5, 625−627.

Committee to Assess Health Risks from Exposure to Low Levels of Ionizing Radiation, 2006. Health Risks From Exposure to Low Levels of Ionizing Radiation: BEIR VII Phase 2. National Academy Press, Washington, DC.

Dom, G., Tarabichi, M., Unger, K., Thomas, G., Oczko-Wojciechowska, M., Bogdanova, T., et al., 2012. A gene expression signature distinguishes normal tissues of sporadic and radiation-induced papillary thyroid carcinomas. BJC 107, 994−1000.

Fenton, C., Anderson, J., Lukes, Y., Dinauer, C.A., Tuttle, R.M., Francis, G.L., 1999. Ras mutations are uncommon in sporadic thyroid cancer in children and young adults. J. Endocrinol. Invest. 22 (10), 781−789.

Fenton, C.L., Lukes, Y., Nicholson, D., Dinauer, C.A., Francis, G.L., Tuttle, R.M., 2000. The ret/PTC mutations are common in sporadic papillary thyroid carcinomas of children and adolescents. J. Clin. Endocrinol. Metab. 85, 1170−1175.

Francis, G.L., Waguespack, S.G., Bauer, A.J., Angelos, P., Benvenga, S., Cerutti, J.M., et al., 2015. Management guidelines for children with thyroid nodules and differentiated thyroid cancer. Thyroid 25 (7), 716−759.

Fugazzola, L., Pilotti, S., Pinchera, A., Vorontsova, T.V., Mondellini, P., Bongarzone, I., et al., 1995. Oncogenic rearrangements of the *RET* proto-oncogene in papillary thyroid carcinomas from children exposed to the chernobyl nuclear accident. Cancer Res. 55, 5617−5620.

Grimwade, D., Ivey, A., Huntly, B.J.P., 2016. Molecular landscape of acute myeloid leukemia in younger adults and its clinical relevance. Blood 127, 29−41.

Handkiewicz-Junak, D., Swierniak, M., Rusinek, D., Oczko-Wojciechowska, M., Dom, G., Maenhaut, C., et al., 2016. Gene signature of the post-Chernobyl papillary thyroid cancer. Eur. J. Nucl. Med. Mol. Imag. 43 (7), 1267−1277.

Haugen, B.R., Alexander, E.K., Bible, K.C., Doherty, G.M., Mandel, S.J., Nikiforov, Y.E., et al., 2016. 2015 American thyroid association management guidelines for adult patients with thyroid nodules and differentiated thyroid cancer: the American thyroid association guidelines task force on thyroid nodules and differentiated thyroid cancer. Thyroid 26 (1), 1−133.

Hess, J., Thomas, G.A., Bauer, V., Bogdanova, T., Wienberg, J., Zitzelsberger, H., et al., 2011. Gain of chromosome band 7q11 in papillary thyroid carcinomas of young patients is associated with exposure to low dose irradiation. PNAS 108, 9595−9600.

Hieber, L., Huber, R., Bauer, V., Schäffner, Q., Braselmann, H., Thomas, G., et al., 2011. Chromosomal rearrangements in post-Chernobyl papillary thyroid carcinomas: evaluation by spectral karyotyping and automated interphase FISH. J. Biomed. Biotechnol. 2011, 693691.

Hillebrandt, S., Streffer, C., Demidchik, E.P., Biko, J., Reiners, C., 1997. Polymorphisms in the p53 gene in thyroid tumours and blood samples of children from areas in Belarus. Mutat. Res. 381 (2), 201−207.

Ito, T., Seyama, T., Mizuno, T., Tsuyama, N., Hayashi, T., Hayashi, Y., et al., 1992. Unique association of p53 mutations with undifferentiated but not with differentiated carcinomas of the thyroid gland. Cancer Res. 52 (5), 1369−1371.

Kaiser, J.C., Meckbach REidemüller, M., Selmansberger, M., Unger, K., Shpak, V., Blettner, M., et al., 2016. Integration of a radiation biomarker into modeling of thyroid carcinogenesis and post-Chernobyl risk assessment. Carcinogenesis 37 (12), 1152–1160.

Kazakov, V.S., Demidchik, E.P., Astakhova, L.N., 1992. Thyroid cancer after Chernobyl. Nature 359, 21.

Kimura, E.T., Nikiforova, M.N., Zhu, Z., Knauf, J.A., Nikiforov, Y.E., Fagin, J.A., 2003. High prevalence of BRAF mutations in thyroid cancer: genetic evidence for constitutive activation of the RET/PTC-RAS-BRAF signaling pathway in papillary thyroid carcinoma. Cancer Res. 63, 1454–1457.

Klugbauer, S., Lengfelder, E., Demidchik, E.P., Rabes, H.M., 1995. High prevalence of RET rearrangement in thyroid tumours of children from Belarus after the Chernobyl reactor accident. Oncogene 11 (12), 2459–2467.

Kumagai, A., Namba, H., Saenko, V., Ashizawa, K., Ohtsuru, A., Ito, M., et al., 2004. Low Frequency of BRAF^{T1796A}mutations in childhood thyroid cancer. JCEM 89, 4280–4284.

Leeman-Neill, R., Brenner, A.V., Little, M.P., Bogdanova, T.I., Hatch, M., Zurnadzy, L., et al., 2013. RET/PTC and PAX8/PPARγ chromosomal rearrangements in post-Chernobyl thyroid cancer and their association with I-131 radiation dose and other characteristics. Cancer 119 (10), 1792–1799.

Leeman-Neill, R., Kelly, L., Liu, P., Brenner, A.V., Little, M.P., Bogdanova, T.I., et al., 2014. ETV6-NTRK3 is a common chromosomal rearrangement in radiation-associated thyroid cancer. Cancer 120 (6), 799–807.

Lemoine, N.R., Mayall, E.S., Wyllie, F.S., Williams, E.D., Goyna, M., Stringer, B., et al., 1989. High frequency of ras oncogene activation in all stages of human thyroid tumourigenesis. Oncogene 4 (2), 159–164.

Lima, J., Trovisco, V., Soares, S., Maximo, V., Maghales, J., Salvatore, G., et al., 2004. BRAF mutations are not a major event in post- Chernobyl Thyroid Carcinomas. JCEM 89, 4267–4271.

LiVolsi, V.A., Abrosimov, A.A., Bogdanova, T., Fadda, G., Hunt, J.L., Rosai, J., et al., 2011. The Chernobyl thyroid cancer experience: pathology. Clin. Oncol. 23, 261–267.

McGuire, A., Brown, J.A.L., Malone, C., McLaughlin, R., Kerin, M.J., 2015. Effects of Age on the Detection and Management of Breast Cancer. Cancers (Basel) 7 (2), 908–929.

Muir, C., Waterhouse, J., Mack, T., Powell, J., Whelan, S. IARC Scientific Publications no 88. V. Lyon: International Agency for Research on Cancer; 1987. Cancer incidence in five continents.

Nikiforov, Y.E., Nikiforova, M.N., Gnepp, D.R., Fagin, J.A., 1996. Prevalence of mutations of ras and p53 in benign and malignant thyroid tumours from children exposed to radiation after the Chernobyl nuclear accident. Oncogene 13 (4), 687–693.

Nikiforov, Y.E., Rowland, J.M., Bove, K.E., Monforte-Munoz, H., Fagin, J.A., 1997. Distinct pattern of ret oncogene rearrangements in morphological variants of radiation-induced and sporadic thyroid papillary carcinomas in children. Cancer Res. 57, 1690–1694.

Parma, J., Van Sande, J., Swillens, S., Tonacchera, M., Dumont, J., Vassart, G., 1995. Somatic mutations causing constitutive activity of the thyrotropin receptor are the major cause of hyperfunctioning thyroid adenomas: identification of additional mutations activating both the cyclic adenosine 3',5'-monophosphate and inositol phosphate-Ca2 + cascades. Mol. Endocrinol. 9 (6), 725–733.

Pierotti, M.A., Greco, A., 2006. Oncogenic rearrangements of the NTRK1/NGF receptor. Cancer Lett. 232 (1), 90–98.

Powell, N.G., Jeremiah, J., Morishita, M., Bethel, J., Bogdanova, T., Tronko, M., et al., 2005. Frequency of BRAF T1794A mutation in thyroid papillary carcinoma relates to age of patient at diagnosis and not to radiation exposure. J. Pathol. 205, 558–564.

Rabes, H.M., Demidchik, E.P., Sidorow, J.D., Lengfelder, E., Beimfohr, C., Hoelzel, D., et al., 2000. Pattern of radiation-induced RET and NTRK1 rearrangements in 191 post-chernobyl papillary thyroid carcinomas: biological, phenotypic, and clinical implications. Clin. Cancer Res. 6 (3), 1093–1103.

Ricarte-Filho, J.C., Li, S., Garcia-Rendueles, M.E., Montero-Conde, C., Voza, F., Knauf, J.A., et al., 2013. Identification of kinase fusion oncogenes in post-Chernobyl radiation-induced thyroid cancers. J. Clin. Invest. 123 (11), 4935–4944.

Ron, E., Lubin, J.H., Shore, R.E., Mabuchi, K., Modan, B., Pottern, L.M., et al., 1995. Thyroid cancer after exposure to external radiation: a pooled analysis of seven studies. Radiat. Res. 141, 259–277.

Russo, D., Arturi, F., Schlumberger, M., Caillou, B., Monier, R., Filetti, S., et al., 1995. Activating mutations of the TSH receptor in differentiated thyroid carcinomas. Oncogene 11 (9), 1907–1911.

Santoro, M., Thomas, G.A., Vecchio, G., Williams, G.H., Fusco, A., Chiappetta, G., et al., 2000. Gene rearrangement and Chernobyl related thyroid cancers. BJC 82, 315–322.

Schoetz, U., Saenko, V., Yamashita, S., Thomas, G.A., 2014. Molecular biology studies of Ukrainian thyroid cancer after Chernobyl. In Tronko M, Bogdanova TI, Saenko V, Thomas GA, Likhtarov I, Yamashita S Thyroid Cancer After Chernobyl – dosimetry, epidemiology, pathology, molecular biology. NASHIM143–174.

Selmansberger, M., Kaiser, J.C., Hess, J., Güthlin, D., Likhtarev, I., Shpak, V., et al., 2015a. Dose-dependent expression of CLIP2 in post-Chernobyl papillary thyroid carcinomas. Carcinogenesis 36 (7), 748–756.

Selmansberger, M., Braselmann, M., Hess, J., Bogdanova, T., Abend, M., Tronko, M., et al., 2015b. Genomic copy number analysis of Chernobyl papillary thyroid carcinoma in the Ukrainian-American Cohort. Carcinogenesis 36 (11), 1381–1387.

Smida, J., Zitzelsberger, H., Kellerer, A.M., Lehmann, L., Minkus, G., Negele, T., et al., 1997. p53 mutations in childhood thyroid tumours from Belarus and in thyroid tumours without radiation history. Int. J. Cancer 73 (6), 802–807.

Stein, L., Rothschild, J., Luce, J., Cowell, J.K., Thomas, G., Bogdanova, T.I., et al., 2010. Copy number and gene expression alterations in radiation-induced papillary thyroid carcinoma from chernobyl pediatric patients. Thyroid 20, 475–487.

Suchy, B., Waldmann, V., Klugbauer, S., Rabes, H.M., 1998. Absence of RAS and p53 mutations in thyroid carcinomas of children after Chernobyl in contrast to adult thyroid tumours. Br. J. Cancer 77 (6), 952–955.

Thompson, D., Mabuchi, K., Ron, E., Soda, M., Tokunaga, M., Ochikubo, S., et al., 1994. Cancer incidence in atomic bomb survivors. Part II: Solid tumours, 1958-1987. Radiat. Res. 137, S17-S6.

Unger, K., Zitzelsberger, H., Santoro, M., Salvatore, G., Bogdanova, T.I., Braselmann, H., et al., 2004. Heterogeneity in the distribution of RET/PTC rearrangements within individual post-Chernobyl papillary thyroid carcinomas. JCEM 89, 4272–4279.

Unger, K., Zurnadzhy, L., Walch, A., Mall, M., Bogdanova, T.I., Braselmann, H., et al., 2006. RET rearrangements in post-Chernobyl papillary thyroid carcinomas with a short latency analysed by interphase FISH. BJC 94, 1472–1477.

UNSCEAR report: Exposures and effects of the Chernobyl Accident. Annex J. 2000 http://www.unscear.org/docs/reports/2000/Volume%20II_Effects/AnnexJ_pages%20451-566.pdf.

UNSCEAR report: Health effects due to radiation from the Chernobyl accident. Annex D 2008 http://www.unscear.org/docs/reports/2008/1180076_Report_2008_Annex_D.pdf.

Williams, E.D., Abrosimov, A., Bogdanova, T.I., Demidchik, E.P., LiVolsi, V., Lushnikov, E., et al., 2004. Thyroid carcinoma after chernobyl. Latent period, morphology and aggressivity. BJC 90, 2219–2224.

Williams, E.D., Abrosimov, A., Bogdanova, T., Demidchik, E.P., Ito, M., LiVolsi, V., et al., 2008. Morphologic characteristics of Chernobyl-related childhood papillary thyroid carcinomas are independent of radiation exposure but vary with iodine intake. Thyroid 18, 847–852.

Williams, G.H., Rooney, S., Thomas, G.A., Cummins, G., Williams, E.D., 1996. Ret activation in adult and childhood papillary thyroid carcinoma using a RT-nPCR approach on archival material. BJC 74, 585–589.

Zhu, Z., Ciampi, R., Nikiforova, M.N., Gandhi, M., Nikiforov, Y.E., 2006. Prevalence of *RET/PTC* rearrangements in thyroid papillary carcinomas: effects of the detection methods and genetic heterogeneity. JCEM 91, 3603–3610.

FURTHER READING

Harach, R., Williams, E.D., 1995. Childhood thyroid cancer in England and Wales. BJC 72, 777–783.

Sierk, A.E., Askin, F.B., Reddick, R.L., Thomas, C.G., 1990. Pediatric thyroid cancer. Pediatr. Pathol. 10, 877–893.

PART III

Fukushima + 5

CHAPTER 13

A Review of Studies on Thyroid Dose Estimation After the Fukushima Accident

Tetsuo Ishikawa

Fukushima Medical University, Fukushima, Japan; Hiroshima University, Hiroshima, Japan

INTRODUCTION

Much radioiodine was released into the environment from the Fukushima Daiichi Nuclear Power Plant accident, leading to concern about radiation exposure to the thyroid. Due to the short half-life of ^{131}I, only limited measurements were done for the thyroid and ^{131}I concentrations in air, food, and water. Then, unsolved issues remain for estimation of thyroid equivalent doses. Many efforts have been made to reconstruct these thyroid equivalent doses. This chapter reviews thyroid equivalent doses estimated by international authorities and Japanese research groups.

Hereafter, thyroid equivalent dose and effective dose indicate the doses due to the accident and do not include doses due to natural radiation. For reference, thyroid equivalent dose due to natural radiation is estimated to be 1 mSv/year (UNSCEAR, 2014). Also, thyroid equivalent dose is simply expressed as thyroid dose.

ESTIMATION BY INTERNATIONAL ORGANIZATIONS

The first comprehensive report on dose estimation for Fukushima residents was published by the WHO (World Health Organization) as a "preliminary dose estimation" in May 2012 (WHO, 2012). The report estimated doses using conservative assumptions to avoid any dose underestimation. For example, people in the most highly affected areas outside the 20-km radius continued to live there for 4 months after the accident. Inhalation dose was calculated based on time-integrated radionuclide concentration in air, which was calculated from ground

Thyroid Cancer and Nuclear Accidents. DOI: http://dx.doi.org/10.1016/B978-0-12-812768-1.00013-7

deposition levels. Ingestion dose was estimated based on a food database. Consequently, thyroid dose for the most-affected area (Namie Town) was estimated to be 100–200 mSv for 1-year-old infants. In other affected areas than Namie Town, thyroid dose was estimated to be 10–100 mSv for 1-year-old infants and 10-year-old children (Table 13.1). Following the preliminary dose estimation, WHO published its "health risk assessment" in February 2013 (WHO, 2013). In this report, thyroid dose for the two most-affected areas, Namie Town and Iitate Village, were estimated to be 122 and 73 mSv for 1-year-old infants, respectively.

The United Nations Scientific Committee on Atomic Radiation published the *2013 UNSCEAR Report* in April 2014 (UNSCEAR, 2014). In this report, ingestion doses to the thyroids were estimated based on the FAO/IAEA food database. Inhalation doses were estimated based on radionuclide concentration in air calculated from deposited activity. For evacuated areas, typical evacuation patterns were applied to estimate district average thyroid doses. The *2013 UNSCEAR Report* noted that more information became available after the Committee completed its dose estimations and that the dose estimates might overestimate actual exposures. The thyroid doses for Namie Town, Iitate Village, and other evacuated areas estimated by this report are shown in Table 13.1. Although the doses to the thyroid are expressed as absorbed dose (mGy) in this report, these are shown as thyroid equivalent dose (mSv) in Table 13.1. The thyroid doses estimated by WHO and UNSCEAR included both internal and external doses received for the first year. Exceptions were doses for Namie Town and Iitate Village in the WHO reports. These doses were estimated for the first 4 months.

Following the *2013 UNSCEAR Report*, the UNSCEAR white paper was published in October 2015 (UNSCEAR, 2015). It reviews literature published before the end of December, and comprises a digest of new information and its implications for the *2013 UNSCEAR Report*. However, the thyroid doses shown in the *2013 UNSCEAR Report* were not updated there. Another comprehensive report on doses due to the accident was published by the IAEA (2015). It reviews publications and data available up to March 2015, but does not present its own estimation of thyroid doses.

Table 13.1 A Comparison of Thyroid Doses Estimated by International Organizations and Japanese Research Groups

Source	1-Year-Old Infants (mSv)			10-Year-Old Children (mSv)			Adults (mSv)		
	Namie	Iitate	Other Evacuated Areas	Namie	Iitate	Other Evacuated Areas	Namie	Iitate	Other Evacuated Areas
WHO (2012) Preliminary dose estimation[a]	100–200	10–100	10–100	10–100	10–100	10–100	10–100	10–100	10–100
WHO (2013) Health risk assessment[a]	122	73	35–48	95	52	18–28	63	34	11–17
UNSCEAR (2014)	81–83	56	15–82	58	34	12–55	34–35	21	7–32
Tokonami et al. (2012) (thyroid measurement)[b]	–	–	–	4.2 (n = 8)	–	–	3.5 (n = 54)	–	–
Kim et al. (2015) (thyroid screening)[b]	–	–	–	–	<5 (n = 315)	<5 (n = 765)[c]	–	–	–
Hosoda et al. (2013) (based on WBC)[b]	–	–	–	0.5 (n = 2393)[d]	–	–	–	–	–
Kim et al. (2016c) (based on WBC)[b]	–	–	–	–	–	–	3.5 (n = 90)[d]	3.5 (n=20)[d]	3.5 (n = 64)[d]
Ishikawa et al. (2015), Kamiya et al. (2016) (external dose for the first year[e])	2	6	2	2	6	2	2	6	2

[a]Doses within 20 km of the Fukushima site were not assessed.

[b]Median values for subjects examined (the number of subjects is shown as "n = "), internal dose only.

[c]The number includes subjects from Iwaki City (nonevacuated area, n = 134).

[d]The numbers include both adults and children. The number of adults was larger for the study by Kim et al., whereas that of children was larger for the study by Hosoda et al. (see text).

[e]Median values.

ESTIMATION REPORTED BY JAPANESE RESEARCH GROUPS

Effective doses due to external exposure for Fukushima residents were investigated by a large-scale survey, as described later. Thyroid dose due to external exposure can be estimated from external effective dose. Thus, this section first deals with the survey on effective dose due to external exposure and its conversion to thyroid dose due to external exposure. Then, estimation of thyroid dose due to internal exposure is mentioned and total thyroid dose is discussed from the viewpoint of comparison with estimations by international organizations.

External Dose to Thyroid

The ICRP (2010) publication gives ratios of effective dose to thyroid dose in various irradiation geometries. In a horizontally irradiated geometry (equally from all directions), the ratios are about 1.1−1.2 for gamma rays with energies of 100−800 keV, which indicates that thyroid dose due to external radiation is almost equal to effective dose due to external radiation.

In the "Basic Survey" on external dose estimation targeting all residents in Fukushima Prefecture (Ishikawa et al., 2015), personal behavior data (daily time budget and record of movement for the first 4 months after the accident) were obtained by using questionnaires. The individual effective doses for the first 4 months were estimated by superimposing the behavior data on the gamma ray dose rate maps. Although the overall response rate to the questionnaire was around 27%, that for eight municipalities in evacuated areas exceeded 50% (FMU, 2016). According to the survey results, median effective dose due to external exposure was 0.5 mSv (average: 0.8 mSv) for Soso region, which included most of the evacuated areas. The low dose was due to prompt evacuation from the 20-km zone. For Namie Town, the median was around 1 mSv. However, for Iitate Village (outside the 20-km zone), the median was around 4 mSv due to a delayed evacuation order. The dependence of the effective doses on age groups was not obvious (Ishikawa, 2017).

Several months after the accident, most municipalities in Fukushima Prefecture started individual dose measurements using personal dosimeters that were mainly distributed to children and pregnant women. The effective dose due to external exposure for the first year could be roughly estimated by adding the estimated dose by the basic survey (first 4 months) to a dose multiplied by 8 monthly individual doses estimated using personal dosimeters (Ishikawa, 2017).

After the first 4 months, almost all people in evacuated areas had moved to areas with lower ambient dose. In typical cities where evacuees moved, the median dose for the 8 months could be around 1 mSv (Kamiya et al., 2016).

Considering the basic survey results and personal dosimeter measurements, the median thyroid dose due to external exposure for the first year was estimated at around 2 mSv for most evacuees including Namie Town residents (Table 13.1). For Iitate Village residents, however, the estimated value was around 6 mSv.

Internal Dose to Thyroid Estimated by Human Measurement

Approaches to estimate thyroid dose due to internal exposure are of two types: direct human body measurements and model calculations. The former includes direct measurement of thyroid and estimation of thyroid dose from whole-body counting (WBC) of cesium using an assumed intake ratio of ^{131}I to cesium. The latter is based on a food database for ingestion and reproducing ^{131}I concentration in air by atmospheric simulation for inhalation. Generally, the former would be more reliable, although the subjects were limited. Then, this section reviews human measurement studies, and the next section discusses simulation studies and their limitations.

Tokonami et al. (2012) directly measured thyroid of evacuees using a gamma ray spectrometer which can estimate activity for each radionuclide. Among 62 subjects of Namie Town and Minami-soma City, 42 subjects had detectable ^{131}I amounts. The median and maximum thyroid dose for adults (54 subjects) were 3.5 and 33 mSv, respectively. The median dose reported for children was similar (Table 13.1).

Another data set on direct measurement of thyroid was from screening with survey meters for 1080 children (Kim et al., 2015). The method was based on dose rate measurement without identifying each radionuclide. The median doses for Iitate Village and two other municipalities can be read as <5 mSv from literature graphs (Kim et al., 2015).

On the other hand, two papers were published regarding thyroid dose estimation based on WBC of cesium (Hosoda et al., 2013; Kim et al., 2016c). An advantage of this method is that WBC of cesium has been conducted on a larger scale compared with the thyroid activity measurement.

In the study by Tokonami et al. (2012), ^{134}Cs was measured for some of the 62 subjects, in addition to ^{131}I. Based on these measurements, Hosoda et al. (2013) estimated the intake ratio (^{131}I/^{134}Cs). On the other hand, a total of 2393 residents of Namie Town were examined (around 80% of them were children) by WBC. Among them, 399 residents (children, 252; adults, 147) had detectable amounts of ^{134}Cs and ^{137}Cs. Using the estimated intake ratio (0.9) and WBC data for cesium, the median thyroid dose among those 2393 residents was estimated to be 0.5 mSv (Table 13.1).

Kim et al. (2016c) estimated thyroid doses from WBC results for 174 subjects from evacuated areas (children, 49; adults, 125). Ninety of these subjects resided in Namie Town and 20 were Iitate Village residents. Median and maximum thyroid dose were 3.5 and 32 mSv for adult subjects of Namie Town, respectively, which agreed well with the corresponding values found by Tokonami et al. (Table 13.1). The study also indicates the median for thyroid doses between Namie and non-Namie was almost the same.

Among the estimations based on human measurements, the doses estimated by Hosoda et al. (2013) seem to be lower. This would be because Hosoda et al. used a lower intake ratio (0.9) than Kim et al. (2016c) (3.8). The point needs further study, but Kim et al. (2016a) suggested that a value of 3 is a reasonable representative value.

Internal Dose to Thyroid by Simulation
Since human measurements were limited, estimation of inhalation dose by using atmospheric dispersion models could be a useful method for reconstructing thyroid doses for a large population.

Kim et al. (2015) indicated that doses estimated by simulation correspond to the 90th percentile or more of doses estimated from measurements, which may be because no protective measures were considered in the simulation. For example, ^{131}I concentration indoors was assumed to be the same as that outdoors. If actually taken protective measures and the personal behaviors (daily time budget and evacuation process) are considered, the simulation results may approach the doses estimated from measurements. Also, updating the atmospheric simulation and dose contribution from short-lived radio-nuclides such as ^{132}Te and ^{132}I are unfinished issues, which may affect the dose estimation by simulation (Ishikawa, 2017).

In addition, the atmospheric dispersion models do not consider dose from ingestion. Thyroid dose from ingestion is a controversial issue (Ishikawa, 2017; Kim et al., 2016b). Thyroid dose due to inhalation seems to be consistent between the *2013 UNSCEAR Report* and the study by Kim et al (2016b). On the other hand, UNSCEAR estimated thyroid dose (1-year-old infants) due to ingestion as 33 mSv even for nonevacuated areas, although Kim et al. (2016c) suggested that dose from ingestion is trivial from a comparison between their measurements with later WBC. A survey on food provided in evacuation centers supports this suggestion (Ishikawa, 2017).

Total Thyroid Dose and its Comparison With Estimation by Other Studies

As described above, dose estimation by simulation tends to give over-estimated results at present. Then, total thyroid dose was estimated by combining thyroid dose due to internal exposure by human measurements with thyroid dose due to external exposure.

As an example, for Namie Town adults, median thyroid dose due to internal exposure could be <5 mSv and that due to external exposure for the first year could be around 2 mSv, which would result in a total dose of <10 mSv. For Iitate Village, the median thyroid dose due to external exposure for the first year could be around 6 mSv. Considering internal dose reported (Table 13.1), the median of total thyroid dose could be around 10 mSv for adults. However, it should be noted that thyroid doses for children and infants would be larger than those for adults, especially for internal exposure, as can be seen in estimations by UNSCEAR and WHO.

Also, it should be noted that doses could be distributed in a wide range. The maximum dose estimated from WBC was estimated to be 84 mSv (Kim et al., 2016c), although it was an outlier. As the IAEA (2015) report suggested, distribution of individual doses can be approximated by log-normal distribution in some cases. The distribution of individual thyroid doses also could be the same, with a long tail on the side of higher doses.

SUMMARY

Thyroid doses to Fukushima residents estimated by human measurements and model calculations were reviewed. The doses estimated in model calculations by international authorities tended to be higher than estimations from human measurements. Based on human measurements, the median doses for the two most-affected areas, Namie Town and Iitate Village, could be around 10 mSv or less for adults, including external exposure. However, it should be noted that doses would be distributed in a wide range and that thyroid doses for children and infants would be larger than those for adults. Efforts continue to be made to reconstruct the whole picture of thyroid doses to Fukushima residents.

REFERENCES

FMU (Fukushima Medical University), 2016. Proceedings of the 24th Fukushima Oversight Committee Meeting. Available at: http://fmu-global.jp/2016/09/15/proceedings-of-the-24th-prefectural-oversight-committee-meeting-for-fukushima-health-management-survey/ Accessed November 30, 2016.

Hosoda, M., Tokonami, S., Akiba, S., Kurihara, O., Sorimachi, A., Ishikawa, T., et al., 2013. Estimation of internal exposure of the thyroid to ^{131}I on the basis of [134]Cs accumulated in the body among evacuees of the Fukushima Daiichi Nuclear Power Station accident. Environ. Int. 61, 73–76.

IAEA (International Atomic Energy Agency), 2015. The Fukushima Daiichi Accident: Technical Volume 4/5 Radiological Consequences. International Atomic Energy Agency, Vienna.

ICRP (International Commission on Radiological Protection), 2010. Conversion Coefficients for Radiological Protection Quantities for External Radiation Exposures. ICRP Publication 116, Ann. ICRP 40, pp. 2–5.

Ishikawa, T., 2016. Radiation doses and associated risk from the Fukushima nuclear accident-a review of recent publications. Asia Pacif. J. Public Health 29 (2S), 18S–28S.

Ishikawa, T., Yasumura, S., Ozasa, K., Kobashi, G., Yasuda, H., Miyazaki, M., et al., 2015. The Fukushima health management survey: estimation of external doses to residents in Fukushima Prefecture. Sci Rep 5, 12712.

Kamiya, K., Ishikawa, T., Yasumura, S., Sakai, A., Ohira, T., Takahashi, H., et al., 2016. External and internal exposure to Fukushima residents. Radiat. Prot. Dosim. 171, 7–13.

Kim, E., Tani, K., Kunishima, N., Kurihara, O., Sakai, K., Akashi, M., 2015. Estimation of early internal doses to Fukushima residents after the nuclear disaster based on the atmospheric dispersion simulation. Radiat Prot Dosim, Advanced Access published August 30, 2015.

Kim, E., Kurihara, O., Tani, K., Ohmachi, Y., Fukutsu, K., Sakai, K., et al., 2016a. Intake ratio of ^{131}I to ^{137}Cs derived from thyroid and whole-body doses to Fukushima residents. Radiat. Prot. Dosim. 168 (3), 408–418.

Kim, E., Kurihara, O., Kunishima, N., Momose, T., Ishikawa, T., Akashi, M., 2016b. Internal thyroid doses to Fukushima residents —estimation and issues remaining. J. Radiat. Res. 57 (S1), i118–i126.

Kim, E., Kurihara, O., Kunishima, N., Kunishima, N., Nakano, T., Tani, K., et al., 2016c. Early intake of radiocesium by residents living near the TEPCO Fukushima Dai-ichi Nuclear Power Plant after the accident. Part 1: internal doses based on whole-body measurements by NIRS. Health Phys. 115 (5), 451–464.

Tokonami, S., Hosoda, M., Akiba, S., Sorimachi, A., Kashiwakura, I., Balonov, M., 2012. Thyroid doses for evacuees from the Fukushima nuclear accident. Sci. Rep. 2, 507.

UNSCEAR (United Nations Scientific Committee on the Effects of Atomic Radiation), 2014. UNSCEAR 2013 Report Annex A: Levels and Effects of Radiation Exposure due to the Nuclear Accident After the 2011 Great East-Japan Earthquake and Tsunami. United Nations, New York.

UNSCEAR (United Nations Scientific Committee on the Effects of Atomic Radiation), 2015. Developments Since the 2013 UNSCEAR Report on the Levels and Effects of Radiation Exposure due to the Nuclear Accident Following the Great East-Japan Earthquake and Tsunami. A 2015 White Paper to Guide the Scientific Committee's Future Program of Work. United Nations, New York.

WHO (World Health Organization), 2012. Preliminary Dose Estimation From the Nuclear Accident After the 2011 Great East Japan Earthquake and Tsunami. World Health Organization, Geneva.

WHO (World Health Organization), 2013. Health Risk Assessment From the Nuclear Accident After the 2011 Great East Japan Earthquake and Tsunami Based on a Preliminary Dose Estimation. World Health Organization, Geneva.

CHAPTER 14

Five-Year Interim Report of Thyroid Ultrasound Examinations in the Fukushima Health Management Survey

Akira Ohtsuru[1], Sanae Midorikawa[1], Satoru Suzuki[1], Hiroki Shimura[1], Takashi Matsuzuka[1] and Shunichi Yamashita[2]

[1]Fukushima Medical University, Fukushima, Japan [2]Nagasaki University, Nagasaki, Japan

BACKGROUND

The Great East Japan Earthquake and Fukushima Daiichi Nuclear Power Plant accident of March 2011 caused concern about the various direct and indirect health impacts of the compound radiation disaster, such as prolonged displacement and dispersion of radioactive material in the environment in affected areas (Hasegawa et al., 2015). The Japanese general public became particularly concerned about the possibility of increased risk of childhood thyroid cancer, similar to that observed following the Chernobyl nuclear accident. The radiation exposure level in Fukushima has been shown to be much lower than that in Chernobyl; however, it was necessary to conduct surveys for both scientific and social purposes (Yamashita and Suzuki, 2013; Ohtsuru et al., 2015). Thus, to mitigate health risks and promote healthy daily living, it was decided to communicate health-related information and establish a system to support residents through health examinations. For this reason, Fukushima Medical University has been conducting thyroid ultrasound examinations as part of the Fukushima Health Management Survey, commissioned by Fukushima Prefecture (Yasumura et al., 2012; Yamashita, 2014).

INTERIM REPORT OF FIRST- AND SECOND-ROUND THYROID ULTRASOUND EXAMINATIONS

The thyroid examination program consists of two stages: the primary examination focuses mainly on nodules and cysts using thyroid ultrasound examination; the confirmatory examination is for individuals

Thyroid Cancer and Nuclear Accidents. DOI: http://dx.doi.org/10.1016/B978-0-12-812768-1.00014-9

who may need detailed follow-up for such lesions (Suzuki et al., 2016a). According to data up to March 2016 (Proceeding of the 23rd Prefectural Oversight Committee Meeting for Fukushima Health Management Survey, 2016), the participation rate in the preliminary baseline survey, first-round thyroid examination in fiscal year (FY) 2011 to FY2013 was 81.7% (300,476 of 367,672 children aged up to 18 years at the time of the disaster). The results of the primary examination are classified into categories A, B, and C. Categories B and C include subjects for which further examination is recommended; and confirmatory examination is not recommended for category A. Category A is subdivided into categories A2 (small cyst less than 20.0 mm or small nodule less than 5 mm in diameter) and A1 (no cysts and no nodules). Category A accounted for 99.2% of the subjects; categories B and C accounted for the remaining 0.8%. With category A, 51.5% of subjects were in A1 and 47.8% in A2. Size distribution of thyroid cysts using ultrasound examination showed that 81.4% were less than 3 mm in diameter, 18.6% were more than 3.1 mm and less than 20.0 mm, and only 0.004% were more than 20.0 mm in diameter. The examination of thyroid nodules indicated that 43.0% were less than 5.0 mm in diameter, 40.3% were more than 5.1 mm and less than 10.0 mm, 13.8% were more than 10.1 mm and less than 20.0 mm, and 3.0% were more than 20.1 mm in diameter. In category A2, 98.8% were cysts; in category B, 99.5% were nodules. The confirmatory examination indicated that 34% of category B subjects should be reclassified as category A. This means that some of the nodules of category B decreased in size and fell under the threshold criteria about 6 months until confirmatory examination. Among category B subjects who underwent fine-needle aspiration cytology, 116 individuals were diagnosed with malignancy or suspected malignancy. As of March 2016, 102 individuals had undergone surgery. The results of postoperative pathological diagnosis were as follows: papillary thyroid cancer, 100 cases; poorly differentiated cancer, one case; and benign nodule, one case.

The scope of subjects for the second-round thyroid examination (first full-scale survey) in FY2014 and FY2015 was expanded to include participants who were born up to April 1, 2012, resulting in about 381,000 subjects (Proceedings of the 24th Prefectural Oversight Committee Meeting for Fukushima Health Management Survey, 2016). The participation rate was 70.2%; category A subjects accounted for 99.2%, and categories B and C accounted for 0.8%. Confirmatory examinations are currently in progress; they have demonstrated that 47% of category B subjects in the first-round examination (preliminary baseline survey) should be reclassified as category A in the second-round examination (first full-scaled survey). As of March 2016, 57 individuals were diagnosed with malignancy or suspected malignancy; 34 subjects had undergone surgery. The results of postoperative pathological diagnosis were as follows: papillary thyroid cancer, 33 cases; and other thyroid tumor. The mean age at diagnosis did not change appreciably between the two round examinations: it was 17.3 ± 2.7 years in the first and 16.8 ± 2.7 years in the second round. The sex ratio was 39:77 (female 66%) in the first and 25:34 (female 58%) in the second round. The mean tumor size was 13.9 ± 7.8 (range, $5.1-45.0$) mm in diameter in the first- and 10.4 ± 5.6 (range, $5.3-35.6$) mm in diameter in the second-round examination. The number of detected thyroid cancer cases was age dependent: the number increased with greater age in both the first- and second-round thyroid examinations. In the early phase of the Chernobyl accident, the increased number of thyroid cancer cases was predominantly among younger children, especially those aged $0-4$ years at the time of the accident; thus, the age distribution we observed was completely different (Wiliams, 2015; Takamura et al., 2016). Therefore, it can be concluded that the lesions identified during the two cycles of the examination over the past 5 years represent the natural incidence in a young population when ultrasound screening is used as a detection methodology.

DOSE ESTIMATION AND THYROID CANCER DETECTION IN THE EARLY PHASE AFTER THE ACCIDENT

Following the Chernobyl accident, the mean thyroid doses of affected children were estimated to be 1548 mGy (preschool children evacuees) and 449 mGy (preschool children living in contaminated areas) (UNSCEAR, 2010 (2008 report)). By contrast, following the Fukushima accident, doses of less than 15 mSv in 99% of children aged $0-14$ years were reported among over 1000 children from some areas suspected of relatively high inhalation exposure (Nagataki and Takamura, 2016). In a report in which thyroid doses were measured for 62 subjects from the evacuation zone, the median equivalent dose was 3.6 mSv in adults and 4.2 mSv in children. Another study using whole-body counting showed that 25% of 196 examinees who stayed in the evacuating or indoor sheltering zone had detectable iodine-131 activity. The median thyroid equivalent dose was 0.67 mSv in the group detecting radioactive iodine. Although the number of direct thyroid dose measurements was limited, those low levels of thyroid doses in Fukushima are unlikely to have produced a detectable excess in thyroid cancer incidence within 4 years after possible exposure (UNSCEAR 2013 report). According to a basic survey of external exposure estimation during the first 4 months after the Fukushima accident (Ishikawa et al., 2015), the maximum exposure level among malignant and suspected malignant cases was 2.1 mSv (Suzuki et al., 2016b).

An ecological study is not appropriate for assessing the radiological health consequences under the very low exposure circumstances or short latent period; however, we have compared the childhood thyroid cancer prevalence in three areas just in case, based on the estimated external dose of a basic survey conducted by the Fukushima Health Management Survey (Ohira et al., 2016). We divided areas into three groups based on individual external doses: $\geq 1\%$ of 5 mSv; $<99\%$ of 1 mSv/year; and other. By means of logistic regression models adjusted for age and sex, we calculated the odds ratios (ORs). Compared with the lowest-dose area as reference, age-, and sex-adjusted ORs (95% confidence intervals) for the highest- and intermediate-dose areas were 1.49 (0.36−6.23) and 1.00 (0.67−1.50), respectively. We then evaluated the ORs for thyroid cancer according to location group using the first-year thyroid doses estimated by the World Health Organization. Compared with the lowest-dose area, age- and sex-adjusted ORs for the highest- and intermediate-thyroid dose areas were 1.50 (0.37−6.15) and 1.01 (0.69−1.47), respectively. Furthermore, we calculated the ORs for thyroid cancer for individual external doses of 1−2 mSv and 2 mSv or more, using the external dose of less than 1 mSv as reference. We found no significant association with the prevalence of thyroid cancer in any dose range.

CANCER DRIVER GENE MUTATION PROFILE

A high proportion (35%−60%) of post-Chernobyl thyroid carcinomas in children possessing RET proto-oncogene rearrangement as a driver mutation were found accompanied by specific pathological features such as follicular variant and solid variant type papillary carcinoma (Thomas et al., 1999; Leeman-Neill et al., 2013). Conversely, point mutation type BRAF and RAS is less frequent. Mitsutake et al. (2015) reported the presence of driver mutations in thyroid cancers treated by surgical operation through the screening detection in the Fukushima Health Management Survey. Among 61 classic papillary thyroid carcinomas (PTCs), including two follicular variant PTCs and four cribriform-morular variant PTCs, and one poorly differentiated thyroid carcinoma; they identified BRAFV600E in 43 cases (63.2%); RET/PTC1 in six cases (8.8%); RET/PTC3 in one case (1.5%); and ETV6/NTRK3 in four cases (5.9%). These driver mutation profiles and the pathological features were completely different from the post-Chernobyl radiation-induced PTCs. The molecular profile of these tumors is what would be predicted from other studies of sporadic thyroid cancer in a similar age group. Taken together with the lack of thyroid cancers in the youngest members of the population in Fukushima this further points to the nonradiogenic etiology of these cancers in Fukushima. The prevalence of the BRAFV600E mutation in Fukushima children was similar to the observations among sporadic adults.

THYROID CANCER SCREENING AND POTENTIAL OVERDIAGNOSIS

Several reports have described dramatic increases over recent decades in the incidence of thyroid cancer, predominantly small papillary carcinoma—even though thyroid cancer-related mortality rates have not changed substantially (Vaccarella et al., 2016). Notably in South Korea, the thyroid cancer incidence in 2011 was 15 times higher than the rate in 1993 (Ahn et al., 2014). Furuya-Kanamori et al. (2016) undertook a search using a fixed-effects meta-analysis model among 35 studies conducted between 1949 and 2007, and 12,834 autopsies. The prevalence of differentiated thyroid carcinoma among the whole examination subgroup was 11.2% (95% confidence interval, 6.7%−16.1%). When the authors applied intensiveness of autopsy thyroid examination to the regression model, the prevalence OR stabilized from 1970. The recent increasing incidence of thyroid carcinoma is not mirrored by a greater prevalence in autopsy studies; this finding suggests that the current rising incidence most likely reflects progress in diagnostic detection.

In general, it has become technologically possible to make an earlier diagnosis of cancer before signs and symptoms are produced. Cancer encompasses cellular abnormalities with a wide variety of natural courses: some grow extremely rapidly; others develop more slowly; still others stop growing completely; and some even regress (Welch and Black, 2010). Continued adherence to standard guidelines may, however, lead to the danger of overdiagnosis in many diseases, especially with psychosocial aspects among pediatric patients (Coon et al., 2014). Another example of overdiagnosis comes from using biomarkers in urine to conduct mass screening for neuroblastoma in the mid-1980s. It was widely accepted by parents with new babies; the participation rate among newborns in Japan was approximately 90% in 2001 (Katanoda, 2016). However, two studies, one in Germany and one in Canada, showed that the neuroblastoma screening programs did not reduce mortality. The reason for the discrepancy in the results for overseas studies and those in Japan remains unknown; however, the committee recommended to the Japanese Ministry of Health, Labor and Welfare that the neuroblastoma program be discontinued. The Japanese government decided to terminate the neuroblastoma mass screening program by the end of FY2003 (Tsubono and Hisamachi, 2004). This case underlines the necessity to evaluate carefully the effectiveness and disadvantages of a new screening method before and after screening is implemented.

The protocol of the Fukushima Health Management Survey is based on the clinical practice guidelines of the Japan Association of Breast and Thyroid Sonography; it is more conservative than the protocol adopted in South Korea in that further examination is recommended only for nodules larger than 5 mm (Suzuki et al., 2016a). However, the American Thyroid Association has recently updated its clinical guidelines to recommend that generally only nodules more than 10 mm should be evaluated for further examination (Haugen et al., 2016). In the Fukushima Health Management Survey, the average detection rate of childhood thyroid cancer is around 0.037% by preliminary baseline survey for the first 3 years of screening (Suzuki et al., 2016b). A similar tendency continues for the following 2 years of screening. The average tumor size of cancer or suspected nodules was 10.4 ± 5.6 (range, 5.3–35.6) mm diameter in second-round examination, suggested that more than 70% of tumors diagnosed malignant or cancer suspected were less than 10 mm diameter. If the outcomes reflect the screening findings, it may be speculated that prevalence will increase further and raise issues of overdiagnosis (Katanoda et al., 2016).

SUMMARY

The relationship between a high prevalence of thyroid cancer and radiation exposure is thought to be very unlikely because of several standpoints; e.g., a limited time interval after the accident, very low doses, age and geographic distributions of thyroid cancer patients, driver mutation patterns, and pathological characteristics. This finding suggests overdiagnosis due to screening effects over the past 5 years. Individual estimates of the thyroid equivalent dose will be required to identify the most vulnerable population in whom the benefits of the screening are greater than any potential harm to individuals and public health dimensions. However, even if the most vulnerable population could be identified from the thyroid dose estimation, the benefits of the screening are thought to be small due to its good prognosis and the lasting psychosocial problem in a lifetime (Midorikawa et al., 2016, 2017). It is further necessary to reconsider screening diagnostic criteria to prevent the risk of overdiagnosis.

REFERENCES

Ahn, H.S., Kim, H.J., Welch, H.G., 2014. Korea's thyroid-cancer "epidemic"—screening and overdiagnosis. N. Engl. J. Med. 371 (19), 1765–1767.

Coon, E.R., Quinonez, R.A., Moyer, V.A., Schroeder, A.R., 2014. Overdiagnosis: how our compulsion for diagnosis may be harming children. Pediatrics 134 (5), 1013–1023.

Furuya-Kanamori, L., Bell, K.J.L., Clark, J., Glasziou, P., Doi, S.A.R., 2016. Prevalence of differentiated thyroid cancer in autopsy studies over six decades: a meta-analysis. J. Clin. Oncol. 34, 3672–3679.

Hasegawa, A., Tanigawa, K., Ohtsuru, A., Yabe, H., Maeda, M., Shigemura, J., et al., 2015. Health effects of radiation and other health problems in the aftermath of nuclear accidents, with an emphasis on Fukushima. Lancet 386, 479–488.

Haugen, B.R., Alexander, E.K., Bible, K.C., Doherty, G.M., Mandel, S.J., Nikiforov, Y.E., et al., 2016. 2015 American Thyroid Association management guidelines for adult patients with thyroid nodules and differentiated thyroid cancer: the American Thyroid Association Guidelines Task Force on Thyroid Nodules and Differentiated Thyroid Cancer. Thyroid 26, 1–133.

Ishikawa, T., Yasumura, S., Ozasa, K., Kobashi, G., Yasuda, H., Miyazaki, M., et al., 2015. The Fukushima Health Management Survey: estimation of external doses to residents in Fukushima Prefecture. Sci. Rep. 5, 12712.

Katanoda, K., 2016. Neuroblastoma mass screening—what can we learn from it? J. Epidemiol. 26 (4), 163–165.

Katanoda, K., Kamo, K., Tsugane, S., 2016. Quantification of the increase in thyroid cancer prevalence in Fukushima after the nuclear disaster in 2011--a potential overdiagnosis? Jpn. J. Clin. Oncol. 46 (3), 284–286.

Leeman-Neill, R.J., Brenner, A.V., Little, M.P., Bogdanova, T.I., Hatch, M., Zurnadzy, L.Y., et al., 2013. RET/PTC and PAX8/PPARγ chromosomal rearrangements in post-Chernobyl thyroid cancer and their association with iodine-131 radiation dose and other characteristics. Cancer 119 (10), 1792−1799.

Midorikawa, S., Suzuki, S., Ohtsuru, A., 2016. After Fukushima: addressing anxiety. Science 352 (6286), 666−667.

Midorikawa, S., Tanigawa, K., Suzuki, S., Ohtsuru, A., 2017. Psychosocial issues related to thyroid examination after radiation disaster. Asia Pacific J. Public Health 29, 63S−73S.

Mitsutake, N., Fukushima, T., Matsuse, M., Rogounovitch, T., Saenko, V., Uchino, S., et al., 2015. BRAF(V600E) mutation is highly prevalent in thyroid carcinomas in the young population in Fukushima: a different oncogenic profile from Chernobyl. Sci. Rep. 5, 16976.

Nagataki, S., Takamura, N., 2016. Radioactive doses—predicted and actual—and likely health effects. Clin. Oncol. (R. Coll. Radiol.) 28, 245−254.

Ohira, T., Takahashi, H., Yasumura, S., Ohtsuru, A., Midorikawa, S., Suzuki, S., et al., 2016. Comparison of childhood thyroid cancer prevalence among 3 areas based on external radiation dose after the Fukushima Daiichi nuclear power plant accident: The Fukushima health management survey. Medicine (Baltimore) 95 (35), e4472.

Ohtsuru, A., Tanigawa, K., Kumagai, A., Niwa, O., Takamura, N., Midorikawa, S., et al., 2015. Nuclear disasters and health: lessons learned, challenges, and proposals. Lancet 386 (9992), 489−497.

Proceeding of the 23rd Prefectural Oversight Committee Meeting for Fukushima Health Management Survey. http://fmu-global.jp/survey/the-23rd-prefectural-oversight-committee-meeting-for-fukushima-health-management-survey/. Accessed December 14, 2016.

Proceedings of the 24th Prefectural Oversight Committee Meeting for Fukushima Health Management Survey. http://fmu-global.jp/survey/the-24th-prefectural-oversight-committee-meeting-for-fukushima-health-managemant-survey/. Accessed December 14, 2016.

Suzuki, S., Suzuki, S., Fukushima, T., Midorikawa, S., Shimura, H., Matsuzuka, T., et al., 2016b. Comprehensive survey results of childhood thyroid ultrasound examinations in Fukushima in the first four years after the Fukushima Daiichi nuclear power plant accident. Thyroid 26 (6), 843−851.

Suzuki, S., Yamashita, S., Fukushima, T., Nakano, K., Midorikawa, S., Ohtsuru, A., et al., 2016a. The protocol and preliminary baseline survey results of the thyroid ultrasound examination in Fukushima [Rapid Communication]. Endocr. J. 63 (3), 315−321.

Takamura, N., Orita, M., Saenko, V., Yamashita, S., Nagataki, S., Demidchik, Y., 2016. Radiation and risk of thyroid cancer: Fukushima and Chernobyl. Lancet Diabetes Endocrinol. 4 (8), 647.

Thomas, G.A., Bunnell, H., Cook, H.A., Williams, E.D., Nerovnya, A., Cherstvoy, E.D., et al., 1999. High prevalence of RET/PTC rearrangements in Ukrainian and Belarussian post-Chernobyl thyroid papillary carcinomas: a strong correlation between RET/PTC3 and the solid-follicular variant. J. Clin. Endocrinol. Metab. 84 (11), 4232−4238.

Tsubono, Y., Hisamichi, S., 2004. A halt to neuroblastoma screening in Japan. N. Engl. J. Med. 350 (19), 2010−2011.

United Nations Scientific Committee on the Effects of Atomic Radiation, 2010. Sources and Effects of Ionizing Radiation: UNSCEAR 2008 Report to the General Assembly With Scientific Annexes. United Nations, New York.

United Nations Scientific Committee on the Effects of Atomic Radiation. Sources and effects of ionizing radiation, 2013. UNSCEAR 2013 Report Volume I. Report to the General Assembly. Scientific Annexes A: Levels and Effects of Radiation Exposure due to the Nuclear Accident After the 2011 Great East-Japan Earthquake and Tsunami. United Nations, New York.

Vaccarella, S., Franceschi, S., Bray, F., Wild, C.P., Plummer, M.I., Dal Maso, L., 2016. Worldwide thyroid-cancer epidemic? The increasing impact of overdiagnosis. N. Engl. J. Med. 375 (7), 614−617.

Welch, H.G., Black, W.C., 2010. Overdiagnosis in cancer. J. Natl. Cancer Inst. 102, 605–613.

Williams, D., 2015. Thyroid growth and cancer. Eur. Thyroid J. 4, 164–173.

Yamashita, S., 2014. Tenth Warren, K Memorial Sinclair keynote address—the Fukushima nuclear power plant accident and comprehensive health risk management. Health Phys. 106, 166–180.

Yamashita, S., Suzuki, S., 2013. Risk of thyroid cancer after the Fukushima nuclear power plant accident. Respir. Investig. 51, 128–133.

Yasumura, S., Hosoya, M., Yamashita, S., Kamiya, K., Abe, M., Akashi, M., et al., 2012. Study protocol for the Fukushima Health Management Survey. J. Epidemiol. 22, 375–383.

CHAPTER 15

The Features of Childhood and Adolescent Thyroid Cancer After the Fukushima Nuclear Power Plant Accident

Shinichi Suzuki

Fukushima Medical University School of Medicine, Fukushima, Japan

INTRODUCTION

After the Fukushima Daiichi Nuclear Power Plant accident that followed the Great East Japan Earthquake and tsunami on March 11, 2011, residents in Fukushima Prefecture faced concerns over possible health effects caused by low-dose radiation exposure.

As there was a significant increase in childhood thyroid carcinoma in Belarus and Ukraine after the Chernobyl nuclear accident in 1986, the Japanese public was particularly concerned about a similar increase in Japan, as a result of the Fukushima accident.

The Japanese government decided to perform thyroid ultrasound examinations (TUE) (Suzuki et al., 2016a,b; Suzuki, 2016) on all children in Fukushima prefecture as one of the four detailed surveys contributing to the Fukushima Health Management Survey (FHMS).

A program of ultrasound examination was initiated for people aged 18 years or younger at the time of the disaster.

This chapter provides information on the features of childhood and adolescent thyroid cancer from the operated cases following the TUE.

RESULTS

TUE (Table 15.1)

The results of the TUE (Suzuki et al., 2016a,b; Suzuki, 2016) are summarized in Table 15.1. In the first-round survey, the preliminary

Thyroid Cancer and Nuclear Accidents. DOI: http://dx.doi.org/10.1016/B978-0-12-812768-1.00015-0

Table 15.1 Summary of the Results of TUE

	Preliminary Baseline Survey (PBLS)	Full-Scale Survey (FSS)
Duration	2011/10/09−2014/03/31[a]	2014/04/01−2016/03/31
No. of primary exams	300,476	267,769
Participation rate	81.7%	70.2%
Category A	298,182 (99.2%)	265,708 (99.2%)
A1/A2	154,607/143,575 (51.5/ 47.8%)	102,870/151,739 (40.1/ 59.1%)
Category B	2293 (0.8%)	2061 (0.8%)
Category C	1 (0.0%)	0 (0.0%)
No. of confirmatory exams	2294	2061
Participation rate	92.8%	65.3%
No. of malignant or suspected malignancy diagnosed by FNAC	116	57
No. of operated cases (cancer/benign tumor)	102 (101/1)	30 (30/0)

[a]2015/4/30 finished (primary exam) 2016/3/31 collected (confirmatory exam).

baseline survey (PBLS), 300,476 subjects (participation rate: 81.7%) were screened by March 31, 2016. Among them, 2294 subjects were recommended for a second screening, in which 116 subjects were diagnosed with malignancy or suspected malignancy by fine-needle aspiration cytology (FNAC) following precise ultrasound examination. A second survey was completed on 267,769 subjects, among them, 2294 subjects were recommended for a second screening, in which 57 were also diagnosed with malignancy by FNAC. Furthermore, a third-round survey started from April, 2016 (Proceedings of the 23rd Prefectural Oversight Committee Meeting for Fukushima Health Management Survey).

Surgical Treatment
Preparation for Surgery After Confirmatory Examination of TUE
Among the 173 subjects (116 from the PBLS and 57 from the second survey) diagnosed with malignancy or suspected malignancy by FNAC, 132 underwent surgery; one benign nodule and 131 thyroid cancers were confirmed. Thirty-nine subjects are still waiting for surgical treatment or selected nonsurgical observation after extensive consultation with their doctors. Of the 131 operated thyroid cancer cases,

125 underwent surgery at our department. Before operation, all cases were examined by neck and lung computed tomography.

Clinical Characteristics of the 125 Thyroid Cancers Operated on in Fukushima Medical University Hospital

Among the 125 cases, the male to female ratio was 44:81 (1:1.8), and the mean age at disaster and at diagnosis were 14.8 and 17.8 years old, respectively. Mean tumor size, which was measured prior to operation by ultrasonography, was 14.0 mm (range 5−53 mm). All cases had a diameter of over 5 mm; our protocol is to wait until a further round of screening in cases where the tumor diameter is less than 5 mm. One hundred and twenty-one (96.8%) tumors were ipsilateral and only four (3.2%) were bilateral. Sixty-eight tumors were in the right lobe, 53 in the left of the thyroid.

Preoperative Staging

Preoperative staging using the TNM classification system was used (www.uicc.org/resources/tnm). This system characterizes tumors on the basis of size (T), the degree of invasion of the tumor into lymph nodes (N), and the presence of distant metastasis (M). The system is used both preoperatively to guide the type of operation performed and post-operatively when the pathologist is able to observe the excised lesion and investigate the extent of invasion by the tumor, at the microscopic level, into neighboring structures (veins, lymph nodes). The majority of the cases were less than 20 mm and restricted to the thyroid (T1). A total of 80.1% of patients were T1 (35.2% T1a and 45.6% T1b). A smaller percentage (9.6%) was between 20 and 40 mm but still con-tained within the thyroid (T2) and a similar number (9.6%) was mini-mally invasive or tumor size >4 cm, limited to the thyroid (T3) (Table 15.2). For extrathyroidal invasion, 90.4% had nothing, 9.6% was minimally invasive (T3), and no cases were widely invasive (T4). Only two cases were over 4 cm and also indicated extrathyroidal mini-mal invasion. The majority of cases examined preoperatively showed no lymph node metastasis (N0; 77.6%); 4% were N1a and 18.4% were N1b. Only three cases (2.4%) showed distant metastases; all had lung metastasis. Two of these cases were male, one was aged 16 years old at the time of the disaster and 19, 18 years old at diagnosis (cT3cN1a, pT3pN1a and cT3cN1b, pT2pN1b respectively). A third was female and aged 10 years old at the disaster and 13 years old at diagnosis (cT1bcN1b, pT3pN1b).

Table 15.2 Pre- and Postoperative TNM Findings (*n* = 125)

	cTNM			pTNM	
cT	1a	44 (35.2%)	pT	1a	43 (34.4%)
	1b	57 (45.6%)		1b	31 (24.8%)
	2	12 (9.6%)		2	2 (1.6%)
	3	12 (9.6%)		3	49 (39.2%)
	4	0		4	0
cN	0	97 (77.6%)	pN	0	28 (22.4%)
	1a	5 (4.0%)		1a	76 (60.8%)
	1b	23 (18.4%)		1b	21 (16.8%)
M	0	122 (97.6%)			
	1	3 (2.4%)[a]			

[a]*M1 cases; 16 years old (19) male with cT3cN1a and pT3pN1a, 16 years old (18) male with cT3cN1b and pT2ppN1b and 10 years old (13) female with cT1bN1b and pT3pEX1 pN1b (age at diagnosis, with age at disaster in parentheses).*

Operation Criteria of Small Tumors Without Invasion or Metastasis (cT1acN0cM0)
Forty-four (35.2%) of the cases classified as T1a were smaller than 10 mm, and had no evidence of invasion or metastasis. Twenty cases were suspected of having extrathyroidal invasion, three cases were suspected to have nodal metastasis, 10 cases were close to recurrent laryngeal nerve (RLN), and seven cases were close to the trachea. In one case there was preexisting Graves disease and a lung tumor. Eleven patients elected not to have thyroid surgery immediately.

Postoperative (Pathological) TNM Findings
In the postoperative TNM classification, 59.2% were T1 (34.4% T1a and 24.8% T1b), 1.6% were classified as T2, and 39.2% were classified as T3. There were no cases classified as T4. The number of cases that were classified as T3 postoperatively (39.2%) was much higher than preoperatively (9.6%). This increase was due to evidence of invasion found on pathological examination of the operative specimen. Postoperatively, all cases showed either no lymph node metastasis (22.4%) or metastasis was limited only to local lymph nodes (60.8% N1a, 16.8% N1b).

Surgical Procedure Used
A total of 91.2% of the subjects underwent hemithyroidectomy or lobectomy, while only 8.8% received total thyroidectomy. All cases underwent lymph node dissection, 17.6% in the lateral zone and 82.4%

in the central area. Of those undergoing lateral neck lymph node dissection, the majority (16%) had lymph nodes dissected on one side only; bilateral dissection was performed in 1.6% of cases. All primary cases were operated by small skin incision, e.g., 3 cm for hemithyroidectomy even with lateral neck lymph node dissection and 4−5 cm for total thyroidectomy with lateral neck dissection. All cases also used intraoperative nerve monitoring system (IONM) to avoid RLN injury.

Complications of Surgery
There was no complication of hypothyroidism except in those cases in which total thyroidectomy was performed and those cases which required levothyroxine supplemented cases prior to surgery due to Hashimoto disease. There were no other complications, e.g., hypoparathyroidism, permanent RLN palsy, or postoperative bleeding. One case had persistent RLN palsy regardless of the use of IONM systems. Although some cases showed elevated TSH level above the upper level of normal, normalized TSH levels were obtained following an iodine-restricted diet.

Histopathological Diagnosis
Papillary thyroid cancer (PTC) was diagnosed in 121 subjects (98%); three subjects were diagnosed with poorly differentiated thyroid carcinomas and one with "other," which was unclassified. One hundred and ten PTC cases were of the classical type; four were of the follicular variant, three of the diffuse sclerosing variant, and four were of the cribriform morula variant, which was related to familial adenomatous polyposis. The solid variant of PTC, which was common after the Chernobyl disaster, was not detected.

Intraglandular spread and calcification were observed in high frequency, 61.6% and 78.4%, respectively.

DISCUSSION

Benign thyroid tumors and cysts are common in the population as a whole, but thyroid cancer is relatively rare. There is a clear association between exposure to radiation and the risk of thyroid cancer, and it is for this reason that the TUE was included as part of the larger FHMS.

In 2012−13 just after the initiation of the TUE, a surprising incidence of thyroid cysts, categorized as A2 lesions in the TUE, was found. Most were cysts without a solid component such as colloid cyst or simple cyst (Suzuki et al., 2016b). Some of the media reported that the incidence of thyroid cysts was rapidly increasing in Fukushima after the disaster, and expressed concern that the increase was due to radiation exposure. To obtain comparative data for these findings in Fukushima, the Ministry of Environment entrusted the Japan Association of Breast and Thyroid Sonology to perform TUE in other areas of Japan using the same protocol as that used in Fukushima Prefecture (Taniguchi et al., 2001; Hayashida et al., 2013). This survey was performed in three prefectures, Aomori, Yamanashi, and Nagasaki. These were located far from Fukushima to provide data on a control population with no known exposure to radiation. The frequency of A2 lesions in Aomori, Yamanashi, and Nagasaki prefectures was 56.5%, higher than that in Fukushima. This suggested that the increased prevalence of thyroid cysts was unrelated to radiation exposure, and was more likely to be due to the use of highly sophisticated ultrasonic screening. The increased frequency in Aomori, Yamanashi, and Nagasaki was also possibly due to the exclusion of those aged under 3 years of age from the screening program in these areas. The prevalence of A2 lesions is known to increase with age. In the FSS (Suzuki et al., 2016b), frequency of A2 lesions was similar to that in the three prefectures, as those now being screened in the FSS phase in Fukushima were aged more than 2 years old.

The attention of the media then focused on what, at the time, seemed an unexpectedly high number of thyroid cancers being detected by the TUE in Fukushima Prefecture. Thyroid cancer occurs at all ages but two out of three thyroid cancers become clinically apparent between the ages of 20 and 55. The early media reports did not take into account the natural incidence of thyroid cancer in the Japanese population and the fact that the ultrasensitive technology used effectively moves the natural incidence curve to the left. In addition, we know that the thyroid gland naturally produces very small cancers, many of which do not become clinically apparent. Screening has the added effect of identifying these cancers too. Both of these factors combine so that it would be expected that more thyroid cancer would be found in the population, just because the screening was carried out. Thyroid cancer screening is rarely carried out in such a young population. It is worth noting that the incidence of 30 cases per 10,000 children and adolescents has now stabilized.

The PTCs identified in the TUE do not appear to differ markedly in respect of their pathology or clinical phenotype to PTCs identified in other populations of a similar age (Enomoto et al., 2012). However, the distribution of the age of the patients at operation is significantly different when compared with the first reports of an increase of thyroid cancer following Chernobyl. In the PBLS, the mean age at diagnosis and at the time of disaster was 17.3 and 14.8 years, respectively; of these, 38 were male and 75 were female (Proceedings of the 23rd Prefectural Oversight Committee Meeting for Fukushima Health Management Survey). There was no case aged below 5 years at the time of the accident. These results arc similar to the results reported by Tronko et al. (2014) in the first 4 years after the Chernobyl accident. It is interesting to note that the age distribution changed dramatically in Ukraine more than 4 years after the accident, with increasing numbers of thyroid cancers in those aged below 5 years at the time of the Chernobyl accident (Enomoto et al., 2012). In the FSS, the age distribution remains as it was for the PBLS, suggesting that the increased frequency of thyroid cancer in Fukushima is unlikely to be due to exposure to radiation, but much more likely to result from increased ascertainment as a result of the TUE.

The treatment pathway for thyroid cancer is defined by the risk that the cancer poses. The majority of the cancers identified in the TUE are not so high risk—confined to the thyroid gland, minimally invasive with either no spread or spread to local lymph nodes only. It is therefore important to balance the benefits of treatment against the risks associated with surgery and adjuvant therapy. Although the majority of data on the treatment of low-and intermediate-risk thyroid cancer comes from adult-onset disease, there is evidence that childhood thyroid cancer, like its adult counterpart, results in a very low rate of mortality. Active surveillance (AS) is recommended for thyroid cancers under 10 mm diameter without suspected invasion or metastasis in the adult, and our protocol recommends adopting the same approach for cancers detected as a result of the TUE (Suzuki et al., 2016b; Suzuki, 2012, 2016). If the tumor is observed to have grown in the following round of screening, an operation may be deemed appropriate at that later time. For low-risk thyroid cancer our protocol is to use conservative surgery, i.e., hemithyroidectomy and prophylactic central neck dissection, and is consistent with Japanese guidelines (Yoshida, 2010). Leboulleux et al. (2016) recommended AS for microPTC. However, our operated cases with a diameter of 5–10 mm were not considered to be suitable for AS as described by Leboulleux et al. (2016).

This contrasts with the total thyroidectomy that was frequently performed in Belarus (Demidchik et al., 2006). In our view, this avoids overtreatment that could result from the use of the TUE and provides the correct balance between risk and benefit.

CONCLUSION

Preliminary and full-scale TUE surveys have been performed on 300,476 and 267,769 children, respectively, since the Fukushima accident 5 years ago. Following use of FNAC 116 patients identified in the PLBS and 57 identified in the FSS were diagnosed with malignant or suspected malignant tumors. Of these, 132 were confirmed as having thyroid cancer after thyroid surgery, and one was confirmed as having a benign nodule as of the end of March 2016. The increase of thyroid cancers in Fukushima after the accident seems to be due to the effects of large-scale screening using highly sophisticated ultrasound examination, and not related to radiation exposure. However, the TUE should be continued long-term to determine whether the frequency of childhood and adolescent thyroid cancer due to exposure to radiation from the Fukushima accident increases or not. The present diagnostic criteria for ultrasound and FNAC as well as the guidelines for surgical treatment must be followed in order to avoid overdiagnosis or overtreatment.

ACKNOWLEDGMENT

The data used on the FHMS was referred from the open-access homepage of Fukushima Radiation and Health at the Radiation Medical Science Center for the FHMS, Fukushima Medical University (http://fmu-global.jp). The author is most grateful to Professor G. Thomas and Professor Shunichi Yamashita for the suggestion and English proofreading of this manuscript. Special appreciation to our colleagues from the Department of Thyroid and Endocrinology, Fukushima Medical University: Satoru Suzuki, Toshihiko Fukushima, Hiroshi Mizunuma, Izumi Nakamura, Keiichi Nakano, Satoshi Suzuki, Chiyo Ookouchi, Mai Ashizawa, Yosuke Tachiya, Takao Takahashi, Tazuko Kawasaki, and Manabu Iwadate. And I thank especially Emeritus Professor of Fukushima Medical University Seiichi Takenoshita for support and encouragement during TUE and treatment of thyroid cancer. I also thank the FHMS Group: Hitoshi Ohto, Masafumi Abe, Koichi Tanigawa, Kenji Kamiya, Seiji Yasumura, Mitsuaki Hosoya, Akira Ohtsuru, Akira Sakai, Hiroki Shimura, Sanae Midorikawa, Takashi Matsuduka, Tetsuya Ohira, Hideto Takahashi, and Yoshimasa

Ohira. And I also express my appreciation to the professors of Nagasaki University, Noboru Takamura, Naomi Hayashida, Norisato Mitsutake, Vladimir Saenko, and the Japanese panels of thyroid experts.

REFERENCES

Demidchik, Y.E., Demidchik, E.P., Reiners, C., Biko, J., Mine, M., Saenko, V.A., et al., 2006. Comprehensive clinical assessment of 740 cases of surgically treated thyroid cancer in children of Belarus. Ann. Surg. 243, 525–532.

Enomoto, Y., Enomoto, K., Uchino, S., Shibuya, H., Watanabe, S., Noguchi, S., 2012. Clinical features, treatment, and long-term outcome of papillary thyroid cancer in children and adolescents without radiation exposure. World J. Surg. 36, 1241–1246.

Hayashida, N., Imaizumi, M., Shimura, H., Okubo, N., Asari, Y., Nigawara, T., et al., 2013. Investigation Committee for the Proportion of Thyroid Ultrasound Findings. Thyroid ultrasound findings in children from three Japanese prefectures: Aomori, Yamanashi and Nagasaki. PLoS One 23, 8–e83220.

Leboulleux, S., Tuttle, R.M., Pacini, F., Schlumberger, M., 2016. Papillary thyroid microcarcinoma: time to shift from surgery to active surveillance? Lancet Diabetes Endocrinol. 4, 933–942.

Proceedings of the 23rd Prefectural Oversight Committee Meeting for Fukushima Health Management Survey. http://fmu-global.jp/2016/06/07/proceedings-of-the-23rd-prefectural-oversight-committee-meeting-for-fukushima-health-management-survey/.

Suzuki, S., 2012. Thyroid ultrasound guidebook for diagnosis and management. In: Japan Association of Breast and Thyroid Sonology Committee for Thyroidal Terminology and Diagnostic Criteria (Ed.), Chapter V: Diagnosis for Thyroid Lesions, 2nd ed. Nankodo [In Japanese], Tokyo, pp. 25–29.

Suzuki, S., 2016. Childhood and adolescent thyroid cancer in Fukushima after the Fukushima Daiichi nuclear power plant accident: 5 years on. Clin. Oncol. (R. Coll. Radiol.) 28, 263–271.

Suzuki, S., Suzuki, S., Fukushima, T., Midorikawa, S., Shimura, H., Matsuzuka, T., et al., 2016a. Comprehensive survey results of childhood thyroid ultrasound examinations in Fukushima in the first four years after the Fukushima Daiichi nuclear power plant accident. Thyroid 26, 843–851.

Suzuki, S., Yamashita, S., Fukushima, T., Nakano, K., Midorikawa, S., Ohtsuru, A., et al., 2016b. The protocol and preliminary baseline survey results of the thyroid ultrasound examination in Fukushima [Rapid Communication]. Endocr. J. 63, 315–321.

Taniguchi, N., Hayashida, N., Shimura, H., Okubo, N., Asari, Y., Nigawara, T., et al., 2001. Investigation committee for the proportion of thyroid ultrasound findings. J. Med. Ultrason. 40, 219–224.

Tronko, M.D., Saenko, V.A., Shpak, V.M., Bogdanova, T.I., Suzuki, S., Yamashita, S., 2014. Age distribution of childhood thyroid cancer patients in Ukraine after Chernobyl and in Fukushima after the TEPCO-Fukushima Daiichi NPP accident. Thyroid 24, 1547–1548.

Yoshida, A., 2010. Treatment of thyroid tumor. Japanese clinical guidelines. In: Takami, H., Ito, Y., Noguchi, H., Yoshida, A., Okamoto, T. (Eds.), Algorithms for Diagnosis and Treatment, Papillary Thyroid Carcinoma. Springer, New York, p. 10).

CHAPTER 16

Psychosocial Impact of the Thyroid Examination of the Fukushima Health Management Survey

Sanae Midorikawa[1], Akira Ohtsuru[1], Satoru Suzuki[1], Koichi Tanigawa[1], Hitoshi Ohto[1], Masafumi Abe[1] and Kenji Kamiya[1,2]

[1]Fukushima Medical University, Fukushima, Japan [2]Hiroshima University, Hiroshima, Japan

THYROID CANCER SCREENING FOLLOWING THE FUKUSHIMA NUCLEAR POWER PLANT ACCIDENT

The thyroid examinations in the Fukushima Health Management Survey were launched in October 2011 (Suzuki et al., 2016a). At that time, both residents and medical professionals were deeply concerned about radiation exposure and the associated health risks, especially radiation-induced thyroid cancer. Many residents underwent thyroid examination owing to concerns and anxieties about radiation exposure and thyroid cancer.

Prior to these ultrasound examinations, it was difficult to sufficiently explain their details and the characteristics of radiation-induced thyroid cancer to residents. There is no official guidance on how such examination results should be interpreted for the general public. Moreover, as this was the first experience with such examinations for almost everyone involved, considerable time elapsed until the examinees were able to accurately comprehend the meaning of their individual results.

In the past, large-scale thyroid cancer screening had been conducted in situations such as the Chernobyl nuclear accident and for children potentially exposed to iodine-131 from the Hanford (WA, USA) nuclear site (Tronko et al., 1999; Demidchik et al., 2007; Kopecky et al., 2005).

Thyroid Cancer and Nuclear Accidents. DOI: http://dx.doi.org/10.1016/B978-0-12-812768-1.00016-2

There was widespread public concern regarding increased incidence of thyroid cancer owing to radiation exposure based on experiences in Chernobyl (Tronko et al., 1999; Demidchik et al., 2007) and among atomic bomb survivors (Preston et al., 2007; Ron et al., 1995). Although individual thyroid dose estimation was limited especially in the first year, radiation exposure in Fukushima was thought to be much lower compared with those previous nuclear disasters (Tokonami et al., 2012). Therefore, thyroid examinations in Fukushima may have been conducted to ensure children's health over the long-term in response to concerns about potential low-dose radiation exposure. Owing to social demands, thyroid examinations were considered indispensable in Fukushima. However, this examination brought not only overdiagnosis, but also various psychosocial problems regarding the screenings. We therefore reevaluated the screening program in terms of principles and in consideration of the situation after a nuclear power plant accident.

POTENTIAL BENEFITS AND HARMS OF THYROID CANCER SCREENING

Principles and Practice of Screening for Disease in 1968 proposed 10 principles, termed "guides to planning case-finding," as listed below (Wilson and Jonner, 1968). The authors emphasized that it is pointless to consider starting any screening program unless all 10 principles can be met. If the principles are met, careful research is needed to measure the balance of benefits and harms, affordability, and the best means of administering the program. Medical professionals and also the general public have tended to consider screening as always the right thing to do focusing on potential benefits with less regard for potential harm. However, from around 1960, it was increasingly recognized that it was necessary to evaluate both the benefits and harms of screening, implement quality-assured programs, and maintain the ethical duty of providing well-balanced information (Raffle and Gray, 2009).

The 10 principles of screening for disease are as follows (Wilson and Jonner, 1968):

1. The condition sought should be an important health problem.
2. There should be an accepted treatment for patients with a recognized disease.

3. Facilities for diagnosis and treatment should be available.
4. There should be a recognizable latent or early symptomatic phase.
5. There should be a suitable test or examination.
6. The test should be acceptable to the population.
7. The natural history of the condition, including development from latent to declared disease, should be adequately understood.
8. There should be an agreed-upon policy on whom to treat as patients.
9. The cost of case finding (including diagnosis and treatment of patients diagnosed) should be economically balanced in relation to possible expenditure on medical care as a whole.
10. Case finding should be a continuing process and not a "once and for all" project.

With respect to thyroid cancer screening, principles 2, 3, 5, and 6 are met: accepted diagnoses and treatments are available for clinical thyroid cancer cases. However, some of the principles are apparently inappropriate for such screening. For example, thyroid cancer generally has a favorable prognosis; thus, it is difficult to state that it is an important health problem (principle 1). Furthermore, the natural history of thyroid cancer detected by screening is inadequately understood; accordingly, there is no agreed policy about whom to treat as patients (principles 7 and 8).

In a recent review by the US Preventive Services Task Force, Harris et al. (2011) identified a different paradigm that was more useful for evaluating proposed screening programs. This gave a balanced approach compared with estimation of benefits and harms of the program. The authors listed a potential benefit if the following were high: (1) probability of an adverse health outcome without screening; (2) degree to which screening identifies all individuals who would suffer the adverse health outcome; and (3) magnitude of incremental health benefit of earlier versus later treatment as a result of screening. Conversely, Harris et al. (2011) recognized that the following are important as potential harms: (1) frequency of false-positive screening tests and experience of individuals with false-positive results; (2) frequency of overdiagnosis and experience of people who are overdiagnosed; and (3) frequency and severity of harms of workup and treatment.

Potential benefits are considered to be few from the following standpoints. First, thyroid cancer has excellent prognosis without screening; according to the Guideline of the American Thyroid Association, thyroid cancer screening is not recommended worldwide (Haugen et al., 2015). The probability of an adverse health outcome without screening would appear to be very low, and there is a very low possibility of benefits for an adult. Second, with each screened case, it is difficult to determine clinically whether thyroid cancer may advance or remain latent; however, very few patients begin suffering from advanced thyroid cancer. Thus, the possibility of any benefits may be small at that point. Third, there is no evidence that cases diagnosed through screening have better prognoses (Ahn et al., 2014).

Potential harms are seen as substantial from two standpoints. First, thyroid nodules are frequently found in the thyroid gland using ultrasound examination, and most cases are benign and indolent (Kwong et al., 2015). Thyroid cancer screening produces many false-positive results. People receiving false-positive results suffer an unnecessary negative experience rather than a sense of security from knowing that they do not have cancer. These outcomes should be considered potential harms in terms of medical examinations of asymptomatic individuals. Second, considerable evidence points to the danger of overdiagnosis in thyroid cancer screening using ultrasound (Welch and Black, 2010); patients who are overdiagnosed undergo adverse psychological experiences (Lee et al., 2016). The greater the degree of overdiagnosis, the greater is the negative experience on the part of the patient. Such factors likely represent major harms in thyroid cancer screening. Third, the diagnostic procedures in thyroid cancer screening are not generally invasive except fine-needle aspiration cytology. So, this third point is not considered to represent a harmful factor.

Owing to the few potential benefits and substantial potential harms, thyroid cancer screening programs have not been recommended. If there is unavoidable need to launch a screening program, an evidence-based protocol must be prepared and sufficiently explained to residents before the program starts.

ISSUES OF THYROID ULTRASOUND EXAMINATIONS IN THE FUKUSHIMA HEALTH MANAGEMENT SURVEY

Next, we reevaluated the thyroid examinations in Fukushima under the chaotic situation following the nuclear power plant accident. Some possible benefits of the thyroid examinations in Fukushima may be considered. First, anxiety about thyroid cancer should diminish when examinees receive normal test results. That certainly seems to have been the case in Fukushima. However, contrary to expectations, even though some results may not have presented clinical problems, such as thyroid cysts, the examinees were not necessarily relieved (Midorikawa, 2014). Second, it is possible to obtain scientific evidence regarding radiation exposure and health risks through thyroid examinations. The evidence obtained from this survey may be meaningful to the lives of residents in the distant future. Examinees should therefore be informed that the benefits of the examination may not be immediate or directly apply to themselves.

Importantly, the potential harms in thyroid cancer screening programs, such as overdiagnosis, false positives, and the related negative experience, may emerge under certain circumstances following a nuclear power plant accident. Almost all the thyroid cancer cases would not have been detected without ultrasound screening; this suggests that the detected cases also included ones of overdiagnosis (Welch and Black, 2010; Katanoda et al., 2016). Residents tend to associate thyroid cancer with radiation exposure; however, in any particular patient, it is difficult to determine clinically whether thyroid cancer is actually related to radiation exposure. Thyroid cancer patients face problems concerning radiation exposure in their long-term futures; as a result, their families (especially mothers of young children) may feel guilt over a long period. This is significant as a harmful outcome of overdiagnosis (Ohtsuru et al., 2015). It has been reported that 0.8% of subjects who underwent thyroid ultrasound examination in Fukushima were determined to be category B, which meant that they required further examinations (Suzuki et al., 2016a). Further, 95% of category B cases were diagnosed as not having thyroid cancer: they were thus false positives. With such category B cases, the examinees and their parents were deeply concerned about the examination results. Even with benign cases, examinees and their families would have been concerned about the cause of disease and had doubts about the relationship to radiation exposure.

Owing to the results of the screening, including overdiagnosis, the reported number of thyroid cancer cases following thyroid examinations in Fukushima was much higher than the figures reported in cancer registries elsewhere in Japan (Suzuki et al., 2016b; Katanoda et al., 2016). However, concerns about the relationship to radiation exposure have persisted deeply among residents, who have been influenced by information they read in newspapers and on the Internet. It is difficult for residents to judge such information scientifically, which renders them susceptible to misplaced fears of thyroid cancer based on screening results.

ADDRESSING PSYCHOSOCIAL ISSUES ARISING FROM THYROID EXAMINATIONS IN FUKUSHIMA

To address the problems detailed above, we have conducted the following efforts among Fukushima residents over the past 5 years: (1) communication with mothers (explanatory meetings); (2) immediate postexamination individual counseling; and (3) class dialogue in schools.

1. The purpose of the explanatory meetings we have given is to reduce parents' anxiety about thyroid cysts, provide information about the postdisaster thyroid examinations, disseminate knowledge about thyroid cancer, and help interpret the results. Hino et al. (2016) have reported on the validity of these meetings for participants. However, the total number of participants was about 8000; low compared with the number of all examinees, which was over 300,000, and that of their family members, which was more than double that number. Many residents still have doubts and anxieties over the purpose of the thyroid examinations, the health risks due to radiation exposure, and interpretation of thyroid cancer screening results.
2. We initiated immediate postexamination individual counseling in October 2014 in the examination venues in response to individual concerns and anxiety. We presented ultrasound images, explained the meaning of findings, and answered questions about radiation exposure and health risks (Midorikawa et al., 2016). There is inadequacy in that we are unable to provide this counseling to many more examinees of school age who are unaccompanied by their parents because such counseling is regarded as a kind of school examination.
3. To provide a better understanding of the purpose of thyroid examinations and interpretation of the results, we have held classes since

2015 about the examinations for elementary to high school students (Midorikawa et al., 2016). We explain the nature of thyroid cysts and that most nodules are not serious and need not be treated. We also discuss thyroid cancer (its symptoms, treatment, and prognosis) and the association between various health risks and diseases including those other than cancer. Through response cards after the classes, we recognized that the students appeared to understand the scientific basis of the medical issues. However, there was also evidence of unexpressed health concerns about daily life following the compound radiation disaster and a vague feeling of unease about the future (Midorikawa et al., 2017).

The above strategies alone are insufficient for fully removing possible harm. To minimize such harm, there is an urgent need to directly reduce the high rates of overdiagnosis and false-positive results.

CHALLENGES FOR MAKING THYROID EXAMINATIONS ACCEPTABLE TO RESIDENTS, AND FUTURE PERSPECTIVES

Following a nuclear disaster, residents tend to have greater concern about radiation exposure and health risks than about the potential harms of screening programs. Moreover, the subjects in the Fukushima screening program were only aged up to 18 years as of March 11, 2011, so they could not have been expected to be aware of the complex reasons behind thyroid examinations and the public perceptions of risk. However, many schoolchildren have taken part, which largely reflects the parents' concerns. There is an ethical dilemma in whether school-age children, who are unable to make decisions autonomously, should be allowed to participate in thyroid examinations that could lead to thyroid cancer diagnosis. We therefore should promote truly voluntary participation in the survey by providing sufficient scientific information, rather than having subjects motivated by fear of radiation exposure or thyroid cancer. Needless to say, we need to provide thorough explanation about individual and epidemiological results of the screening in a manner easily understandable and acceptable to postdisaster citizens. Moreover, while respecting the children's thoughts, we have to confirm the subjects' willingness to undergo screening by providing sufficient information about the meaning of the screening and its potential harms and benefits.

As discussed, it is generally inappropriate to screen for thyroid cancer because the screening will not necessarily result in decreased mortality (Ahn et al., 2014). It is also necessary to reconsider how to conduct thyroid cancer screening after a nuclear accident because of exaggeration of potential harms. Thyroid cancer screening should be limited to the subjects scientifically verified as needing it after evaluating radiation exposure dose and acquiring consent to participate. These collective efforts will reduce potential harms of thyroid cancer screening.

REFERENCES

Ahn, H.S., Kim, H.J., Welch, H.G., 2014. Korea's thyroid-cancer "epidemic"—screening and overdiagnosis. N. Engl. J. Med. 371, 1765–1767.

Demidchik, Y.E., Saenko, V.A., Yamashita, S., 2007. Childhood thyroid cancer in Belarus, Russia and Ukraine after Chernobyl and at present. Arq Bras Endocrinol. Metabol. 51, 748–762.

Harris, R., Sawaya, G.F., Moyer, V.A., Calonge, N., 2011. Reconsidering the criteria for evaluating proposed screening program: reflections from 4 current and former members of the U.S. preventive services. Epidemiol. Rev. 33, 20–35.

Haugen, B.R., Alexander, E.K., Bible, K.C., Doherty, G.M., Mandel, S.J., Nikiforov, Y.E., et al., 2015. American Thyroid Association management guidelines for adult patients with thyroid nodules and differentiated thyroid cancer: The American Thyroid Association Guidelines Task Force on Thyroid Nodules and Differentiated Thyroid Cancer. Thyroid 26, 1–133.

Hino, Y., Murakami, M., Midorikawa, S., Ohtsuru, A., Suzuki, S., Tsuboi, K., et al., 2016. Explanatory meetings on thyroid examination for the "Fukushima Health Management Survey" after the Great East Japan Earthquake: reduction of anxiety and improvement of comprehension. Tohoku J. Exp. Med. 239, 333–343.

Katanoda, K., Kamo, K., Tsugane, S., 2016. Quantification of the increase in thyroid cancer prevalence in Fukushima after the nuclear disaster in 2011—a potential overdiagnosis? Jpn. J. Clin. Oncol. 46, 284–286.

Kopecky, K.J., Onstad, L., Hamilton, T.E., Davis, S., 2005. Thyroid ultrasound abnormalities in persons exposed during childhood to ^{131}I from Hanford nuclear site. Thyroid 15, 604–614.

Kwong, N., Medici, M., Angell, T.E., Liu, X., Marqusee, E.S., Cibas, E.S., et al., 2015. The influence of patient age on thyroid nodule formation, multinodularity, and thyroid cancer risk. J. Clin. Endocrinol. Metab. 100, 4434–4440.

Lee, S., Lee, Y.Y., Yoon, H.J., Choi, E., Suh, M., Park, B., et al., 2016. Response to overdiagnosis in thyroid cancer screening among Korean women. Cancer Res. Treat. 48, 883–891.

Midorikawa, S., 2014. Fukushima Report: From the thyroid screening site. Jpn. Med. J. 4723, 16–17 (in Japanese).

Midorikawa, S., Suzuki, S., Ohtsuru, A., 2016. After Fukushima: addressing anxiety. Science. 352, 666–667.

Midorikawa, S., Tanigawa, K., Suzuki, S., Ohtsuru, A., 2017. Psychosocial issues related to thyroid examination after a radiation disaster. Asia Pacific J. Public Health. 29, 63S–73S.

Ohtsuru, A., Tanigawa, K., Kumagai, A., Niwa, O., Takamura, N., Midorikawa, S., et al., 2015. Nuclear disasters and health: lessons learned, challenges, and proposals. Lancet 386, 489–497.

Preston, D.L., Ron, E., Tokuoka, S., Funamoto, S., Nishi, N., Soda, M., et al., 2007. Solid cancer incidence in atomic bomb survivors: 1958-1998. Radiat. Res. 168, 1–64.

Raffle, A., Gray, M., 2009. Screening: Evidence and Practice, 2nd ed. Oxford University Press, Oxford.

Ron, E., Lubin, J.H., Shore, R.E., Mabuchi, K., Modan, B., Pottern, L.M., 1995. Thyroid cancer after exposure to external radiation, a pooled analysis of 7 studies. Radiat. Res. 141, 259–277.

Suzuki, S., Suzuki, S., Fukushima, T., Midorikawa, S., Shimura, H., Matsuzuka, T., et al., 2016b. Comprehensive survey results of childhood thyroid ultrasound examinations in Fukushima in the first four years after the Fukushima Daiichi nuclear power plant accident. Thyroid 26, 843–851.

Suzuki, S., Yamashita, S., Fukushima, T., Nakano, K., Midorikawa, S., Ohtsuru, A., et al., 2016a. The protocol and preliminary baseline survey results of the thyroid ultrasound examination in Fukushima. Endocr. J. 31, 315–321.

Tokonami, S., Hosoda, M., Akiba, S., Sorimachi, A., Kashiwakura, I., Balonov, M., 2012. Thyroid doses for evacuees from the Fukushima nuclear accident. Sci. Rep. 2, 507.

Tronko, M.D., Bogdanova, T.I., Komissarenko, I.V., Epstein, O.V., Oliynyk, V., Kovalenko, A., et al., 1999. Thyroid carcinoma in children and adolescents in Ukraine after the Chernobyl nuclear accident: statistical data and clinicomorphologic characteristics. Cancer 86, 149–156.

Welch, H.G., Black, W.C., 2010. Overdiagnosis in cancer. J. Natl. Cancer Inst. 102, 605–613.

Wilson, J.M.G., Jonner, G., 1968. Principles and Practice of Screening for Disease. World Health Organization, Geneva.

CHAPTER 17

Thyroid Cancer Screening and Overdiagnosis in Korea

Hyeong-Sik Ahn and Hyun-Jung Kim
Korea University, Seoul, Korea

INCREASING INCIDENCE OF THYROID CANCER

Thyroid cancer is the most common carcinoma in the endocrine system, with papillary and follicular carcinomas being the most predominant subtype. While many studies report a recent increase in the incidence of thyroid cancer worldwide (Pellegriti et al., 2013; Vaccarella et al., 2016), its interpretation remains controversial. Some argue that the increase is attributed to increased detection with use of diagnostic technologies (Vigneri et al., 2015), while others point to lifestyle and environmental changes as potential contributors (Almquist et al., 2011; Hodgson et al., 2004; Kilfoy et al., 2011; Kitahara et al., 2011; Mack et al., 2003; Peterson et al., 2012; Zhang et al., 2008).

In many countries, thyroid cancer has become one of the most common cancers among females (Davies and Welch, 2006). Most patients undergo surgery if thyroid cancer is detected, and increased rates of thyroid cancer incidence have raised an important socioeconomic issue.

While the increase in thyroid cancer incidence is a worldwide phenomenon (Burke et al., 2005), Korea has experienced the fastest growth pattern in incidence compared to any other country (Ahn et al., 2014). In this chapter, we describe the relationship between thyroid cancer screening incidence to understand the mechanisms that lie behind the increasing incidence of thyroid cancer in Korea and worldwide.

Thyroid Cancer and Nuclear Accidents. DOI: http://dx.doi.org/10.1016/B978-0-12-812768-1.00017-4

THYROID NODULES AND THYROID CANCER

Studies on fine-needle aspiration cytology (FNAC) or pathology report that thyroid cancer is detected in 3%–10% of patients who present with thyroid nodules. The prevalence of thyroid nodules increases with age and thyroid cancers are more frequently found in larger thyroid nodules than in those of a smaller size (Kitahara et al., 2011). When a thyroid nodule is found, patients often undergo thyroid ultrasonography and subsequently undergo FNAC. FNAC is a primary test for differential diagnosis between a benign and malignant lesion and its sensitivity and specificity are approximately 85% and 90%–95%, respectively.

It is known that performance of ultrasonography-guided FNAC is better than palpation-based FNAC for the detection of thyroid cancer. While palpation-guided FNAC detects thyroid cancer in 1%–10% of nodules, ultrasound-guided biopsy detects thyroid cancer in 7%–22% of nodules (Brito et al., 2013). In a Korean study, it has been reported that approximately 50% of the population have thyroid nodules and among these 5%–10% are subsequently diagnosed with thyroid cancer (Suk et al., 2006; Table 17.1).

EVIDENCE FOR THE INCREASED INCIDENCE OF THYROID CANCER BEING A RESULT OF INCREASED DETECTION

Tumor Size and Histological Characteristics

In studies reporting on thyroid cancer, most of the increase is restricted to an increase in small-sized (0–1.0 cm) papillary carcinoma. In the United States, a rapid increase has been observed between 1998 and 2002 in the incidence of papillary thyroid carcinomas of 0–1.0 cm

Table 17.1 Evidence That the Increasing Incidence of Thyroid Cancer Is due to Increased Detection
1. Increased use of ultrasonography, fine-needle aspiration cytology
2. Increased incidence of small-sized papillary cancer
3. Detection of thyroid cancer from autopsy studies
4. Association between thyroid cancer screening and incidence
5. Increase in coincidental detection of small-sized papillary cancer in diagnostic studies for other diseases

diameter. It is reported that 25% of patients diagnosed with thyroid cancer have tumors less than 1.0 cm in size. Some studies report that thyroid carcinomas were found in 4.2% of the nodules smaller than 1 cm and in 7.4% of the nodules larger than 1 cm (Davies et al., 2010; Tomimori et al., 1995; Yim et al., 2002).

Ultrasound-guided FNAC studies have contributed in detecting smaller-sized nodules and microcarcinoma (Chung, 2008). Until 20 years ago, the common method for thyroid cancer detection was through palpation of the neck, inspection of visible lumps in the throat, or physical examination of asymptomatic patients. With the introduction of ultrasonography in the 1980s, and adoption of ultrasound-guided FNAC in the late 1990s, nodules smaller than 2 cm are regularly subject to diagnostic biopsy (Ezzat et al., 1994). Increased ability to detect small thyroid cancers has increased its clinical significance. Recent guidelines do not recommend active treatment, including surgery for nodules that measure under 1.0 cm in diameter.

Papillary thyroid cancer accounts for 90% of the increase of thyroid cancer as a whole. The incidence of papillary thyroid carcinoma increased remarkably from 1973 to 2002, while other types such as follicular carcinoma, medullary carcinoma, or other malignant tumors remained stable. Because papillary carcinoma does not significantly affect the health or survival of patients, the rise in papillary cancer incidence has raised the issue of overdiagnosis (Ahn et al., 2014; Brito et al., 2013; Lee and Shin, 2014). As mortality is low, an increase in the diagnosis of papillary microcarcinoma subsequently brings more harm than good and has no effect on mortality. However, the overdiagnosis of papillary cancer has the potential to cause harmful effects to the individual patient such as psychological stress, unnecessary surgery, and/or financial burden.

Adoption of Medical Technology

Evidence shows that the increase in thyroid cancer diagnosis is due to the adoption of new imaging technologies. A significant number of patients with thyroid cancer are detected during the evaluation process of thyroid nodules with ultrasonography (Brander et al., 1991, 1992; Cronan, 2008). Thyroid nodules are discovered in around 16% of patients undergoing CT or MRI scans of the neck, and three-quarters of these were found to be less than 1.5 cm in size (Davies and Welch, 2006). Chest CTs performed for study of pulmonary disease, such as obstructive pulmonary thromboembolism, have also resulted in increased detection of thyroid cancer. The number of thyroid biopsies tripled from 1995 to 2005 as a result of the increase in brain MRI scans for cervical radiculopathy evaluation, resulting in increased detection of thyroid nodules by approximately 2.4-fold. The incidences of thyroid cancer were higher in those areas with more endocrinologists and more ultrasound devices per population (Brito et al., 2013; Udelsman and Zhang, 2014).

In the United States, the use of CT scanning tripled between 1995 and 2005, with 173 scans being carried out per 1000 persons. The use of MRI scanning more than doubled during the same period, with 547 scans per 1000 persons.

Improved Access to Healthcare Services
Improved access to healthcare services, including access to new scanning modalities has also contributed to the increase in thyroid cancer. An analysis of 18 regions in the United States showed a significant association between better access to healthcare and a high incidence of papillary thyroid cancer. The incidence of thyroid cancer was higher in higher socioeconomic regions. For instance, in Wisconsin in the United States, as health insurance coverage increased by 5%, the incidence in the state was increased by an average of 1.4 cases of thyroid cancer per 10,000 persons. In a study from 1980 to 2004, the incidence of thyroid cancer increased by 0.5 cases per 10,000 persons, when the average urban income increased to 10,000 dollars. Regions with a higher proportion of university graduates are also associated with an increased incidence of thyroid cancer (Kilfoy et al., 2011).

Autopsy Studies
A series of autopsy studies have reported the existence of asymptomatic papillary thyroid carcinoma. Studies reported that thyroid nodules are found in 49%−57% of deceased people, who had had no clinical symptoms of thyroid cancer during their lives (Vanderlaan, 1947).

Some studies reported prevalence of thyroid cancer at approximately 36%, most of these were occult and smaller than 2−3 mm. Another study reported that asymptomatic thyroid cancer was found in one-third of the people, who died of causes other than thyroid cancer. Most of the cancers found through autopsy studies were asymptomatic papillary thyroid carcinomas sized less than 1 mm. It has also been reported that the prevalence was higher in people who have a history of cervical irradiation; however, there was no similar association with the prevalence of thyroid nodules. Small lesions would be easy to miss if the specimen was sliced at wide intervals, e.g., 2−3 mm (Vanderlaan, 1947).

Nomenclature

Giving a new name to the disease may prevent overdiagnosis and can provide a chance for watchful surveillance rather than surgery for thyroid cancer. Examples of such changes are from "well-differentiated liposarcoma" to "atypical lipomatous tumor," from "class 1 transitional bladder cancer" to "papillary neoplasm of the bladder with low likelihood of malignancy," and from "cervical cancer" to "neoplasm of cervical intraepithelium." In 2016, a group of pathologists has suggested a nomenclature change of "EFVPTC (encapsulated follicular variant of papillary thyroid carcinoma)" to "NIFTP (noninvasive follicular thyroid neoplasm with papillary-like nuclear features)" (Nikiforov et al., 2016). This means that the name of a lesion previous recognized as being a small thyroid cancer has been changed to one implying that the lesion is benign. The newly named NIFTP is said to comprise 10%−20% of total thyroid cancer.

THYROID CANCER INCIDENCE AND OVERDIAGNOSIS IN KOREA

Thyroid Cancer Screening Program in Korea

The Korean government introduced the National Cancer Screening and Health Checkup Programs in 1999 (Ahn et al., 2014), which included screening for breast, colon, gastric, and liver cancer that was free of charge or with a minimum copayment. Though thyroid cancer is not included in the National Cancer Screening Program, many healthcare providers offered an add-on screening service including ultrasonography of the thyroid. Many healthcare institutions as well as primary care clinics are equipped with ultrasonographic devices and thyroid cancer screening services are provided at a price of USD 30−50 (Ahn et al., 2014).

Thyroid Cancer Incidence and Screening

While the incidence of thyroid cancer increased slightly during the 1990s, there was an abrupt jump in thyroid cancer incidence in Korea after 1999 when the national cancer screening program began (Brito et al., 2016). The age-adjusted incidence of thyroid cancer increased by 15-fold between 1993 and 2011. Most of this increase was due to the detection of papillary carcinoma. In contrast to the exponential growth in the incidence of thyroid cancer, mortality from the disease remains almost at the same level.

There was large variation in the incidence of thyroid across the administrative regions in Korea. To assess whether the variation is explained by screening rate in the regions, we analyzed regional screening data from the 2010 Community Health Survey (200,000 respondents across the country). This asked adults aged over 19 whether they received thyroid cancer screening during the past 2 years. The regional screening rates were compared with the incidence of thyroid cancer across different regions in 2008 and 2009, extracted from the national cancer registry data (Ahn et al., 2016). Age- and gender-stratified analyses demonstrated a strong correlation between screening and incidence of thyroid cancer in both genders ($P<.05$) (Fig. 17.1).

Thyroid cancer is a common female cancer in Korea today, with over 40,000 diagnoses in 2011. Most patients diagnosed with thyroid cancer are treated surgically with two-thirds undergoing total thyroidectomy and one-third partial thyroidectomy. According to one study in one institution, the proportion of surgery for tumors less than 1 cm in diameter increased from 14% in 1995 to 56% in 2005. Several practitioners do not follow the clinical practice guidance recommending not to perform biopsy or surgery on tumors less than 0.5 cm. Patients who undergo thyroidectomy for thyroid cancer have to receive thyroid hormone therapy for the rest of their lives and some experience complications or adverse events. In summary, Korea has experienced overdiagnosis of thyroid cancer for over 18 years, mainly due to the increased availability of thyroid ultrasonographic screening.

Thyroid Cancer in Areas Near Nuclear Power Plants

Due to the controversy regarding possible increases in thyroid cancer near nuclear power plants in Korea, a study supported by the Korean government was performed to examine the incidence of cancers in

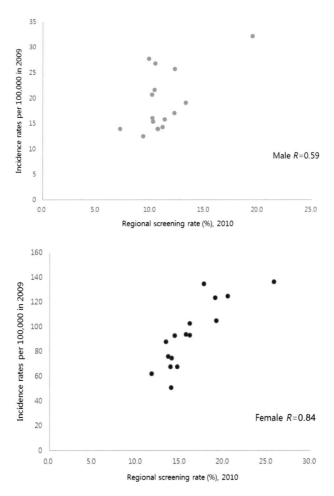

Figure 17.1 Rates of thyroid cancer screening and incidence of thyroid cancer across regions in Korea in male (top) and female adults (bottom).

people residing near to nuclear power plant sites from 1992 to 2011. The results of the study suggested an increased incidence of thyroid cancer around the sites close to nuclear plants. However, controversies still existed whether radiation from nuclear plants was the cause of the increased rates of thyroid cancer, as the study did not control main confounders such as use of detection techniques including ultrasound screening. The nature of this increase, whether or not it is related to radiation, remains to be determined.

In 2015, a study investigated whether there is increased thyroid cancer screening and incidence among residents living in the vicinity of four nuclear sites. The survey was performed for those living in a zone near to the nuclear site, and those living in a remote area as a control. Four nuclear sites and three control sites was selected for the survey.

While increase thyroid cancer incidence was observed in people living in the vicinity of the four nuclear sites, they also performed more diagnostic testing using thyroid ultrasonography. There was an association between thyroid cancer screening and incidence in the regions. Also, the cause for increased thyroid cancer was unlikely to involve radiation exposures, because official estimates for radiation doses from these facilities were too low to explain any causal relationship. The study concludes widespread screening leads to an increased ascertainment of thyroid cancers among people living near to the nuclear sites. This case also demonstrated the effect of thyroid screening on thyroid cancer incidence in Korea.

CONCLUSION

There has been an increased incidence of thyroid cancer worldwide, especially small-sized papillary cancer. The possible cause of such a phenomenon may be due to an increase in detection (i.e., ascertainment) rather than a real increase. Given the wider penetration of advanced medical technologies including ultrasonography and FNAC, an increase restricted to carcinomas of small size and an increase of asymptomatic thyroid cancers identified at autopsy, the increased frequency of thyroid cancer has resulted from increased ascertainment, i.e., an increase in the ability to detect subclinical disease. In Korea, the abrupt increase of thyroid cancer incidence during 15 years is associated with the increased use of screening technologies. Despite the continuous increase, mortality from thyroid cancer has not changed and remains around 0.5 cases per 100,000 persons. This suggests that detecting thyroid cancers early using sensitive screening methods does not have the associated clinical benefits with respect to mortality, and may in other respects do more harm than good.

REFERENCES

Ahn, H.S., Kim, H.J., Welch, H.G., 2014. Korea's thyroid-cancer "epidemic"-screening and over-diagnosis. N. Engl. J. Med. 371 (19), 1765–1767.

Ahn, H.S., Kim, H.J., Kim, K.H., et al., 2016. Thyroid cancer screening in South Korea increases detection of papillary cancers with no impact on other subtypes or thyroid cancer mortality. Thyroid 26 (11), 1535–1540.

Almquist, M., Johansen, D., Bjorge, T., et al., 2011. Metabolic factors and risk of thyroid cancer in the Metabolic syndrome and Cancer project (Me-Can). Cancer Cause Control 22 (5), 743–751.

Brander, A., Viikinkoski, P., Nickels, J., Kivisaari, L., 1991. Thyroid-gland-ultrasound screening in a random adult-population. Radiology 181 (3), 683–687.

Brander, A., Viikinkoski, P., Tuuhea, J., Voutilainen, L., Kivisaari, L., 1992. Clinical versus ultrasound examination of the thyroid-gland in common clinical-practice. J. Clin. Ultrasound. 20 (1), 37–42.

Brito, J.P., Kim, H.J., Han, S.J., Lee, Y.S., Ahn, H.S., 2016. Geographic distribution and evolution of thyroid cancer epidemic in South Korea. Thyroid 26 (6), 864–865.

Brito, J.P., Morris, J.C., Montori, V.M., 2013. Thyroid cancer: zealous imaging has increased detection and treatment of low risk tumours. BMJ 347, f4706.

Brito, J.P., Yarur, A.J., Prokop, L.J., McIver, B., Murad, M.H., Montori, V.M., 2013. Prevalence of thyroid cancer in multinodular goiter versus single nodule: a systematic review and meta-analysis. Thyroid 23 (4), 449–455.

Burke, J.P., Hay, I.D., Dignan, R., et al., 2005. Long-term trends in thyroid carcinoma: a population-based study in Olmsted County, Minnesota, 1935–1999. Mayo Clin. Proc. 80 (6), 753–758.

Chung, J.H., 2008. Prevalence of thyroid nodules detected by ultrasonography in adults for health check-up and analysis of fine needle aspiration cytology. Korean Soc. Endocrinol. 23 (6), 391–394.

Cronan, J.J., 2008. Thyroid nodules: Is it time to turn off the US machines? Radiology 247 (3), 602–604.

Davies, L., Ouellette, M., Hunter, M., Welch, H.G., 2010. The increasing incidence of small thyroid cancers: where are the cases coming from? Laryngoscope 120 (12), 2446–2451.

Davies, L., Welch, H.G., 2006. Increasing incidence of thyroid cancer in the United States, 1973-2002. JAMA 295 (18), 2164–2167.

Ezzat, S., Sarti, D.A., Cain, D.R., Braunstein, G.D., 1994. Thyroid incidentalomas-prevalence by palpation and ultrasonography. Arch. Intern. Med. 154 (16), 1838–1840.

Hodgson, N.C., Button, J., Solorzano, C.C., 2004. Thyroid cancer: is the incidence still increasing? Ann. Surg. Oncol. 11 (12), 1093–1097.

Kilfoy, B.A., Zhang, Y.W., Park, Y., et al., 2011. Dietary nitrate and nitrite and the risk of thyroid cancer in the NIH-AARP Diet and Health Study. Int. J. Cancer 129 (1), 160–172.

Kitahara, C.M., Platz, E.A., Freeman, L.E.B., et al., 2011. Obesity and thyroid cancer risk among US men and women: a pooled analysis of five prospective studies. Cancer Epidem. Biomar. 20 (3), 464–472.

Lee, J.H., Shin, S.W., 2014. Overdiagnosis and screening for thyroid cancer in Korea. Lancet 384 (9957), 1848.

Mack, W.J., Preston-Martin, S., Dal Maso, L., et al., 2003. A pooled analysis of case-control studies of thyroid cancer: cigarette smoking and consumption of alcohol, coffee, and tea. Cancer Cause Control 14 (8), 773–785.

Nikiforov, Y.E., Seethala, R.R., Tallini, G., et al., 2016. Nomenclature revision for encapsulated follicular variant of papillary thyroid carcinoma a paradigm shift to reduce overtreatment of indolent tumors. Jama Oncol. 2 (8), 1023–1029.

Pellegriti, G., Frasca, F., Regalbuto, C., Squatrito, S., Vigneri, R., 2013. Worldwide increasing incidence of thyroid cancer: update on epidemiology and risk factors. J. Cancer Epidemiol.965212.

Peterson, E., De, P., Nuttall, R., 2012. BMI, diet and female reproductive factors as risks for thyroid cancer: a systematic review. PLoS One 7 (1), e29177.

Suk, J.H.K.T., Kim, M.K., Kim, W.B., Kim, H.K., Jeon, S.H., Shong, Y.K., 2006. Prevalence of ultrasonographically-detected thyroid nodules in adults without previous history of thyroid disease. J. Korean Soc. Endocrinol. 21, 389–393.

Tomimori, E., Pedrinola, F., Cavaliere, H., Knobel, M., Medeirosneto, G., 1995. Prevalence of incidental thyroid-disease in a relatively low iodine intake area. Thyroid 5 (4), 273–276.

Udelsman, R., Zhang, Y.W., 2014. The epidemic of thyroid cancer in the United States: the role of endocrinologists and ultrasounds. Thyroid 24 (3), 472–479.

Vaccarella, S., Franceschi, S., Bray, F., Wild, C.P., Plummer, M., Dal Maso, L., 2016. Worldwide thyroid-cancer epidemic? The increasing impact of overdiagnosis. N. Engl. J. Med. 375 (7), 614–617.

Vanderlaan, W.P., 1947. The occurrence of carcinoma of the thyroid gland in autopsy material. N. Engl. J. Med. 237 (7), 221–222.

Vigneri, R., Malandrino, P., Vigneri, P., 2015. The changing epidemiology of thyroid cancer: why is incidence increasing? Curr. Opin. Oncol. 27 (1), 1–7.

Yim, C.H.O.H., Chung, H.Y., Han, K.O., Jang, H.C., Yoon, H.K., Han, I.K., et al., 2002. Prevalence of thyroid nodules detected by ultrasonography in womens attending health chechups. J. Korean Soc. Endocrinol. 17, 183–188.

Zhang, Y., Guo, G.L., Han, X., et al., 2008. Do polybrominated diphenyl ethers (PBDEs) increase the risk of thyroid cancer? Biosci. Hypotheses 1 (4), 195–199.

CHAPTER 18

Management of Papillary Thyroid Carcinoma in Japan

Iwao Sugitani
Nippon Medical School, Tokyo, Japan

In Japan, the annual incidence of thyroid cancer is around 15,000 cases, and approximately 1500 patients die from the disease each year. In iodine intake-sufficient countries like Japan, papillary thyroid carcinoma (PTC) accounts for over 90% of all thyroid cancers.

TRADITIONAL MANAGEMENT OF PATIENTS WITH PTC IN JAPAN

The majority of patients with PTC show an excellent prognosis, but conventional policies for the treatment of PTC have differed between countries with regard to the initial extent of thyroidectomy, postoperative adjuvant therapies including radioactive iodine (RAI) and thyroid-stimulating hormone (TSH) suppression, and methods of surveillance. In Japan, patients are usually treated with thyroid-conserving surgery (lobectomy or subtotal thyroidectomy) and followed-up using ultrasonography (US) without postoperative adjuvant therapies. This represents a very different approach from those of Western countries, where the majority of patients are treated with total thyroidectomy and RAI remnant ablation followed by life-long TSH suppression therapy and periodic measurement of thyroglobulin (Tg).

The basis for these controversies has been socioeconomic differences in the medical care environments of Japan and Western countries (Table 18.1). All publications comparing outcomes between patients who underwent total thyroidectomy and those who received lobectomy have been retrospective studies. In 2007, Bilimoria et al. (2007) demonstrated that total thyroidectomy for PTC with a diameter ≥ 1 cm resulted in lower recurrence rates and even improved survival

Thyroid Cancer and Nuclear Accidents. DOI: http://dx.doi.org/10.1016/B978-0-12-812768-1.00018-6

Table 18.1 Differences in SocioEconomic Environments between Western Countries and Japan	
Western Countries	Japan
1. Many countries are in iodine-deficient areas where highly malignant thyroid cancers have been prevalent 2. Postoperative surveillance is conducted mainly by internists or radiologists 3. Ultrasonography has been an exclusive and expensive procedure	1. World-prominent iodine-sufficient country in which low-risk thyroid cancers are prevalent 2. Postoperative surveillance is conducted by surgeons 3. Strict legal restrictions and shortage of infrastructure for use of radioactive iodine 4. Nationwide use of ultrasonography

compared with lobectomy, using the data of 52,173 patients from the National Cancer Database in the United States. Despite the significant impact of this unprecedentedly large sample size, the study design was also a retrospective multicenter database analysis and therefore carried a potential selection bias. The Japanese Clinical Guidelines for the treatment of thyroid tumor published in 2010 (Imai et al., 2010a) concluded that there is insufficient evidence that total thyroidectomy improves disease-free and cause-specific survival (CSS) of patients compared with lobectomy. However, the committee consensus was that total thyroidectomy is recommended for patients evaluated as high-risk.

RISK-ADAPTED MANAGEMENT OF PTC BASED ON RISK-GROUP CLASSIFICATION SYSTEM

Patients with PTC display very favorable survival rates as high as 95% at 10 years after initial therapy. However, some cases exhibit local recurrence or extensive metastasis postoperatively, and a few patients die of the disease. PTC can be classified into two distinctly different types: low-risk cancer for which mortality is almost identical to that predicted by actuarial curves, and high-risk cancer with a high probability of cancer-specific death. These two are biologically different categories, and low-risk cancer generally does not develop into high-risk cancer time-dependently. To differentiate these two groups, several systems of risk-group classification have been proposed. The most popular prognostic factors are local cancer invasion, distant metastasis, and patient age. Those systems classify the great majority of patients (nearly 90%) as low risk with a 1%–2% mortality rate; the remaining minority of patients belong to the high-risk group and show poor prognosis, with a 50%–75% mortality rate at 10 years postoperatively. The use of proper risk-group definitions is useful not only to tailor selective operative interventions and postoperative adjunctive therapies individually, but also to offer rational information to the patient and to determine the appropriate intensity of surveillance for tumor recurrence.

At the Cancer Institute Hospital (CIH), we retrospectively analyzed a total of 604 patients who had undergone initial surgery for PTC >1 cm in diameter between 1976 and 1998. Mean duration of follow-up was 11 years. Multivariate analysis for CSS identified distant metastasis as the only significant risk factor for younger patients (<50 years). For older patients ($\geq$50 years), distant metastasis, massive extrathyroidal invasion (with preoperative recurrent laryngeal nerve palsy, transluminal invasion of the trachea/esophagus), and large nodal metastasis ($\geq$3 cm) were identified as significant factors. From these results, younger patients with distant metastasis and older patients with any of the three factors were defined as high-risk, while all other patients were defined as low-risk. Overall, 106 high-risk patients (18%) and 498 low-risk patients (82%) displayed 10-year CSS rates of 69% and 99%, respectively (Sugitani et al., 2004). From 2005 onward, we adopted our own risk-adapted approach to patients with PTC based on the risk-group classification system. Patients classified into the high-risk group receive total thyroidectomy with adjuvant therapies, while in patients with unilateral low-risk PTC, the extent of thyroidectomy is determined based on the choices of the patient. We recently verified the validity of our risk-group definition and evaluated treatment outcomes for low-risk patients according to the extent of surgery. Of the 1187 patients who underwent initial surgery for PTC (diameter >1 cm) between 1993 and 2010, a total of 967 (82%) were classified as low-risk and showed a 10-year CSS of 99%. Among low-risk patients, 791 (82%) underwent less-than-total thyroidectomy. Ten-year CSS and disease-free survival (DFS) rates did not differ between patients who received total thyroidectomy and less-than-total thyroidectomy (Table 18.2) (Ebina et al., 2014).

In 2010, the Japanese Clinical Guidelines (Imai et al., 2010) adopted risk-adapted management for patients with PTC, and lobectomy was recommended for low-risk T1N0M0 patients. High-risk PTC was defined as a tumor >5 cm in diameter, extrathyroidal extension to the mucosa of the trachea/esophagus, lymph node metastasis $\geq$3 cm, or extension into surrounding organs and distant metastasis at diagnosis. Total thyroidectomy was recommended for patients

Table 18.2 Extent of Thyroidectomy and Outcomes for Low-Risk PTC				
Extent of Thyroidectomy		Less-Than-Total	Total	*P*
n		791 (82%)	176 (18%)	
Recurrence		67 (9%)	12 (7%)	
Ten-year disease-free survival		87%	91%	0.90
Location of recurrence	Lymph node	52 (7%)	11 (6%)	
	Remnant thyroid	4 (0.5%)	0	
	Other neck	6 (0.8%)	1 (0.6%)	
	Distant	32 (4%)	5 (3%)	
Cause-specific death		9 (1%)	2 (1%)	
Ten-year cause-specific survival		99%	99%	0.61

displaying one or more of these characteristics. Other patients were classified as falling within a "gray zone" and the guidelines state that the extent of surgery should be individually determined based on the balance between incidences of surgical complications and prediction of CSS and DFS evaluated on the risk classifications of the individual institution in which the patient is undergoing surgery. According to the 2009 revision of the American Thyroid Association (ATA) guidelines (American Thyroid Association ATA guidelines taskforce on thyroid nodules and differentiated thyroid cancer et al., 2009), the initial surgical procedure should be near-total or total thyroidectomy for patients with thyroid cancer >1 cm in diameter. However, given the accumulated evidence showing excellent survival for patients with low-risk PTC regardless of the extent of thyroidectomy and the lower risk of surgical complications from lobectomy, the 2015 revision of the ATA guidelines (Haugen et al., 2016) included the concept of risk-adapted management and remarked that lobectomy alone may provide sufficient initial treatment for low-risk PTC. In that edition, high-risk PTC was defined as that with tumor diameter >4 cm, gross extrathyroidal extension, or clinically apparent metastatic disease to nodal or distant sites. For those patients, the guidelines stated that the initial surgical procedure should include near-total or total thyroidectomy. On the other hand, for patients with PTC <1 cm without extrathyroidal extension and clinical metastasis, the procedure should be a thyroid lobectomy. For patients with PTC 1–4 cm in diameter without extrathyroidal extension or metastasis, either a bilateral or a unilateral procedure can be selected. After years of debate, treatment policies for PTC in the East and the West have been largely integrated.

MANAGEMENT OF PAPILLARY MICROCARCINOMA

In the last few decades, the incidence of thyroid cancer has continued to increase all over the world. In the United States, Davies and Welch (2006) reported that the incidence of thyroid cancer increased from 3.6 per 100,000 in 1973 to 8.7 per 100,000 in 2002. This has mainly been attributed to the increased detection of small PTCs by more sensitive diagnostic procedures such as US, rather than from true increases in occurrence rates. Indeed, increased detection and surgery of these carcinomas has not resulted in decreases of mortality from thyroid cancer. Debate on the management of these subclinical thyroid cancers is therefore emerging.

Papillary microcarcinoma (PMC) is defined as PTC with a diameter of ≤ 1.0 cm. Many worldwide autopsy series have shown a surprisingly high prevalence of PMC, ranging from 8% to 36% of patients dying from diseases other than thyroid cancer (Furuya-Kanamori et al., 2016). In comparison, the incidence of clinically evident thyroid cancer is known to be only about 0.1%–0.05% in the general population. Those minute cancers are usually thought to remain innocent and asymptomatic throughout the life of the patient. However, patients once diagnosed with PMC had usually received surgical treatment. At CIH, we retrospectively reviewed outcomes for 178 patients who underwent surgery for PMC between 1976 and 1993 to determine prognostic factors. The most significant risk factors were the presence of clinically apparent lymph node metastasis and hoarseness due to recurrent nerve palsy at the time of diagnosis. All four cases of distant metastasis and four cases of cancer-specific death occurred in 30 patients with symptomatic PMC who had either cervical lymphadenopathy >1 cm in diameter or recurrent nerve invasion, or both. On the other hand, neither distant metastasis nor cause-specific death was seen in the remaining 148 patients without those symptoms (Sugitani and Fujimoto, 1999).

Following these results, we started a prospective clinical trial of active surveillance for asymptomatic PMC (T1aN0M0) in 1995. Patients with PMC diagnosed by US-guided fine-needle aspiration cytology were evaluated as to the presence of distant metastasis, clinically apparent lymphadenopathy (>1 cm), or extrathyroidal invasion. Treatment choice (immediate surgery or active surveillance) was conducted in accordance with the informed decision of the patient. In cases of active surveillance, the tumor is surveyed by modalities such as US every 6 or 12 months. We recommend surgery during follow-up if the patient meets the following criteria: (1) change in patient preferences; (2) tumor has grown on the posterior side of the thyroid, near adjacent structures; (3) development of clinically evident lymph node metastasis or distant metastasis; or (4) increased tumor size (Sugitani et al., 2010). Four hundred and six of 452 patients (90%) with asymptomatic PMC have decided to receive active surveillance rather than immediate surgery. After a mean follow-up of 6.5 years (range, 1−22 years), 28 of 515 lesions (5%) have increased in size. However, 467 lesions (91%) have shown no change and 20 lesions (4%) have decreased in size. No patients have developed extrathyroidal invasion or distant metastasis. Four patients who developed apparent nodal metastasis and 18 patients in whom the tumor increased in size eventually underwent surgery, but postoperative courses were favorable.

A similar prospective trial has been underway at Kuma Hospital in Kobe, Japan, since 1993. They recently reported the results of active surveillance performed on 1235 patients. The mean follow-up period was 75 months and tumor enlargement was seen in 4.9% of patients at 5 years and 8.0% at 10 years. They also did not encounter cases showing distant metastasis or extrathyroidal invasion, although lymph node metastasis had developed in 1.7% of patients at 5 years and 3.8% at 10 years (Miyauchi, 2016). These prospective trials following nearly 2000 patients with T1aN0M0 PTC revealed that the vast majority of tumors did not progress during active surveillance and outcomes were not markedly affected by late salvage surgery. As a result, the Japanese Clinical Guidelines (Imai et al., 2010b) adopted the policy of active surveillance for asymptomatic PMC, representing the first such policy in the world. They stated that surgical treatment is indicated for PMC patients with clinical lymph node metastasis on palpation or imaging studies, distant metastasis, or significant extrathyroidal extension. However, patients without these features can be candidates for observation after extensive explanation of the situation and provision of informed consent. The 2015 ATA guidelines (Haugen et al., 2016) have followed that policy and described that an active surveillance management approach can be considered as an alternative to immediate surgery in patients with very low-risk tumors, such as asymptomatic PMCs.

Advances in the accuracy of health check devices and increasing opportunities for cancer screening among healthy subjects have accelerated screening effects and caused the modern issue of overdiagnosis and overtreatment, such as the "thyroid cancer epidemic" in Korea (Ahn et al., 2014). In Japan, we have reached a consensus that no advantages were gained from detecting PMC in mass screenings for the general population. A 2012 guidebook for the US diagnosis of thyroid diseases recommended that even a solid tumor should not be biopsied if 5 mm or smaller. Thus, the increasing incidence of thyroid cancer in Japan has not been particularly marked compared to other countries (Vaccarella et al., 2015).

MANAGEMENT POLICY OF LOW-RISK PTC IN JAPAN

Fujimoto and Sugitani (1998) performed a long-term (35−45 years) follow-up study on patients with intrathyroidal PTC, in an attempt to reveal the natural history of the disease. Among 49 patients who underwent insufficient surgery, only one definitely died of thyroid cancer. As for PTC, "cancer" is sometimes present that has no deleterious effect on the individual throughout their life. Recent guidelines (Imai et al., 2010; Haugen et al., 2016) have tended to set the range of "low-risk" PTC significantly narrower than the CIH risk-group classification system, with much more emphasis on risk of recurrence than on mortality. According to the National Clinical Database in Japan, total thyroidectomy was performed on 40% of patients with differentiated thyroid cancer (DTC) in 2011. The use of recombinant human TSH for RAI ablation was approved in 2009 and the legal upper limit of RAI use for outpatients was elevated to 30 mCi (1110 MBq) in 2010. Miyauchi et al. (2011) demonstrated that serum Tg-doubling time offers an excellent dynamic prognostic marker for patients with PTC who undergo total thyroidectomy. Tyrosine-kinase inhibitors are newly developed medicines for patients with advanced or metastatic DTC, but are currently indicated only for those patients who have undergone total thyroidectomy and have been revealed to be RAI-refractory. These circumstances have led to a rise in total thyroidectomy compared to thyroid-conserving surgery in Japan. However, total thyroidectomy carries a significantly higher risk of operative complications, including recurrent laryngeal nerve palsy and hypoparathyroidism, compared to less-than-total thyroidectomy. In addition, the procedure commits the patient to a lifetime of thyroid hormone-replacement therapy. Total thyroidectomy has not been the first choice of treatments among patients with low-risk PTC in Japan because Japanese pioneers in thyroidology have understood the biological characteristics of the disease and have selected a conservative approach to treatment in an attempt to maintain quality of life for those patients. Such an approach is considered to ultimately reduce the problems of overdiagnosis and overtreatment of low-risk thyroid carcinomas. These messages from our country are affecting and changing attitudes towards this disease worldwide.

ACKNOWLEDGMENT

Dedicated to the memory of my great mentor, Prof. Yoshihide Fujimoto (1926–2016).

REFERENCES

Ahn, H.S., Kim, H.J., Welch, H.G., 2014. Korea's thyroid-cancer "epidemic": screening and overdiagnosis. N. Engl. J. Med. 371, 1765–1767.

American Thyroid Association (ATA) guidelines taskforce on thyroid nodules and differentiated thyroid cancer, Cooper, D.S., Doherty, G.M., Haugen, B.R., Kloos, R.T., Lee, S.L., et al., 2009. Revised American Thyroid Association management guidelines for patients with thyroid nodules and differentiated thyroid cancer. Thyroid 19, 1167–1214.

Bilimoria, K.Y., Bentrem, D.J., Ko, C.Y., Stewart, A.K., Winchester, D.P., Talamonti, M.S., et al., 2007. Extent of surgery affects survival for papillary thyroid cancer. Ann. Surg. 246, 375–384.

Davies, L., Welch, H.G., 2006. Increasing incidence of thyroid cancer in the United States, 1973-2002. JAMA 295, 2164–2167.

Ebina, A., Sugitani, I., Fujimoto, Y., Yamada, K., 2014. Risk-adapted management of papillary thyroid carcinoma according to our own risk group classification system: is thyroid lobectomy the treatment of choice for low-risk patients?. Surgery 156, 1579–1588.

Fujimoto, Y., Sugitani, I., 1998. Postoperative prognosis of intrathyroidal papillary thyroid carcinoma: long-term (35-45 year) follow-up study. Endocr. J. 45, 475–484.

Furuya-Kanamori, L., Bell, K.J., Clark, J., Glasziou, P., Doi, S.A., 2016. Prevalence of differentiated thyroid cancer in autopsy studies over six decades: a meta-analysis. J. Clin. Oncol. 34, 3672–3679.

Haugen, B.R., Alexander, E.K., Bible, K.C., Doherty, G.M., Mandel, S.J., Nikiforov, Y.E., et al., 2016. 2015 American Thyroid Association management guidelines for adult patients with thyroid nodules and differentiated thyroid cancer: the American Thyroid Association guidelines task force on thyroid nodules and differentiated thyroid cancer. Thyroid 26, 1–133.

Imai, T., Kitano, H., Sugitani, I., Wada, N., 2010a. CQ17. Does total (or near total) thyroidectomy improve the prognosis of papillary carcinoma patients compared to lobectomy or lobectomy isthymectomy? In: Takami, H., Ito, Y., Noguchi, H., Yoshida, A., Okamoto, T. (Eds.), Treatment of Thyroid Tumor. Japanese Clinical Guidelines. Springer, Tokyo, pp. 107–110.

Imai, T., Kitano, H., Sugitani, I., Wada, N., 2010b. CQ20. When can papillary microcarcinoma (papillary carcinoma measuring 1 cm or less) be observed without immediate surgery? In: Takami, H., Ito, Y., Noguchi, H., Yoshida, A., Okamoto, T. (Eds.), Treatment of Thyroid Tumor. Japanese Clinical Guidelines. Springer, Tokyo, pp. 119–122.

Miyauchi, A., 2016. Clinical trials of active surveillance of papillary microcarcinoma of the thyroid. World J. Surg. 40, 516–522.

Miyauchi, A., Kudo, T., Miya, A., Kobayashi, K., Ito, Y., Takamura, Y., et al., 2011. Prognostic impact of serum thyroglobulin doubling-time under thyrotropin suppression in patients with papillary thyroid carcinoma who underwent total thyroidectomy. Thyroid 21, 707–716.

Sugitani, I., Fujimoto, Y., 1999. Symptomatic versus asymptomatic papillary thyroid microcarcinoma: a retrospective analysis of surgical outcome and prognostic factors. Endocr. J. 46, 209–216.

Sugitani, I., Kasai, N., Fujimoto, Y., Yanagisawa, A., 2004. A novel classification system for patients with PTC: addition of the new variables of large (3 cm or greater) nodal metastases and reclassification during the follow-up period. Surgery 135, 139–148.

Sugitani, I., Toda, K., Yamada, K., Yamamoto, N., Ikenaga, M., Fujimoto, Y., 2010. Three distinctly different kinds of papillary thyroid microcarcinoma should be recognized: our treatment strategies and outcomes. World J. Surg. 34, 1222–1231.

Vaccarella, S., Dal Maso, L., Laversanne, M., Bray, F., Plummer, M., Franceschi, S., 2015. The impact of diagnostic changes on the rise in thyroid cancer incidence: a population-based study in selected high-resource countries. Thyroid 25, 1127–1136.

PART *IV*

International Report

UNSCEAR Activities Related to the 2011 Fukushima-Daiichi Nuclear Power Station Accident

Malcolm Crick and Jaya Mohan
Secretariat of the United Nations Scientific Committee on the Effects of Atomic Radiation (UNSCEAR), Vienna, Austria

BACKGROUND TO UNSCEAR

Concerned initially about the effects of atomic weapons testing in the atmosphere, the General Assembly of the United Nations established a Scientific Committee on the Effects of Atomic Radiation (UNSCEAR) on December 3, 1955 (Resolution 913 X, 1955). The mandate of the Committee has been to undertake broad assessments of the sources of ionizing radiation and its effects on human health and the environment. Currently composed of 27 Member States of the United Nations, more than 100 scientists attend the annual session of the committee in Vienna, Austria, to review syntheses of data and information gathered from all over the world. The United Nations Environment Programme (UNEP) is organizationally responsible for supporting the Committee and provides its secretariat.

The scientists that constitute delegations of the 27 countries are nominated based on their qualifications, experience, and expertise. It should be noted that the Committee itself is focused on synthesizing scientific evidence. While its work is relevant to application of science and policy, it does not address these issues itself. Rather it strives to be independent and unbiased in its deliberations (UNSCEAR, 2014). Nevertheless, its scientific findings are often used to underpin and/or guide policy, such as in the case of the 1963 partial test ban treaty (UNSCEAR, 1958), international action plans on worker (Action plan for occupational radiation protection), patient (Draft plan of activities on the radiation protection of the environment), and environmental protection (Para 15 of Report of the United Nations Scientific

Thyroid Cancer and Nuclear Accidents. DOI: http://dx.doi.org/10.1016/B978-0-12-812768-1.00019-8

Committee on the Effects of Atomic Radiation to the sixty-eighth session of the General Assembly) and recovery from the accidents at the Chernobyl and Fukushima-Daiichi nuclear power stations. Its strategic objective for the period 2014–19 (Para 15 of Report of the United Nations Scientific Committee on the Effects of Atomic Radiation to the sixty-eighth session of the General Assembly) is to increase awareness and deepen understanding among decision makers, the scientific community, and civil society with regard to levels of exposure to ionizing radiation and the related health and environmental effects as a sound basis for informed decision-making on radiation-related issues.

UNSCEAR 2013 REPORT ON THE LEVELS AND EFFECTS OF EXPOSURE AFTER THE ACCIDENT

Already in May 2011, the Committee had decided to conduct a major 2-year assessment of the levels and effects of radiation exposure from the accident, an endeavor that was endorsed by the United Nations General Assembly. More than 80 scientists from 18 countries worked on this assessment, and the findings were presented to the General Assembly in October 2013. The Report with its scientific annex entitled "Levels and effects of radiation exposure due to the nuclear accident after the 2011 great east-Japan earthquake and tsunami" (subsequently referred to as the UNSCEAR, 2013a report) was published by the United Nations in April 2014. The main focus of the UNSCEAR 2013 Report was on assessing the exposure of various population groups to ionizing radiation resulting from the nuclear accident, and the implied effects in terms of radiation-induced risks for human health and the environment. The population groups considered included residents of Fukushima Prefecture and other prefectures in Japan; and workers, contractors, and others who were engaged in the emergency work at or around the accident site. The environmental assessment addressed marine, freshwater, and terrestrial ecosystems.

The secretariat of UNSCEAR closely coordinated with other leading international organizations working in this area such as the Preparatory Commission for the Comprehensive Nuclear-Test-Ban Organization, the Food and Agriculture Organization of the United Nations, the International Atomic Energy Agency, the World Health Organization, and the World Meteorological Organization.

Some of the key findings of the 2013 Report were as follows:

- the releases of radioactive material to the atmosphere were about 10% of those from the Chernobyl accident;
- exposure to radioiodine finished within the first few months; the focus now is on long-lived radiocesium; exposures in the first year were the highest with ongoing low exposures in later years; external exposure dominates; the highest doses were to evacuees, but protective measures reduced exposures significantly; for most people, the doses they received are comparable with the natural background;
- overall, cancer rates were expected to remain stable; no discernible increase in cancer rates was expected amongst workers; there was no impact on birth and hereditary effects (the doses were too low); for some children who were most exposed early on, there is a theoretical small increased risk of thyroid cancer, however large increases in the numbers of cases like after the Chernobyl accident could be excluded;
- effects on plants and animals in the environment were localized and transient; the highest exposures were in the marine environment.

FOLLOW-UP TO THE 2013 REPORT

Noting that the 2013 Report only covered information that was available up to October 2012, while new, relevant scientific literature on the subject continued to emerge, the Committee reaffirmed its commitment to follow-up on its work on the accident in 2014, by continuing to closely follow scientific research and developments relevant to understanding the radiation exposures and effects of the accident.

A group of experts was established to appraise new publications in the following areas: atmospheric dispersion and source term; marine dispersion and source term; terrestrial and freshwater dispersion; public dose assessment, remediation and countermeasures; worker dose assessment; nonhuman biota impact assessment; and health risk assessment. The main goal was to identify any inconsistencies between scientific research published and the UNSCEAR 2013 Report. The group also conducted ad hoc analyses to help clarify the situation, responded to questions and critiques of the 2013 Report, and assessed an appropriate time to update it. It was planned to publish the results of the appraisal annually as a White Paper, covering literature published up to the end of the previous calendar year.

The first results of the follow-up work were thus published as a 2015 White Paper, in English and Japanese (Developments since the 2013 UNSCEAR, 2015). The 2016 White Paper was also published the following year (Developments since the 2013 UNSCEAR, 2016), and work on the 2017 edition is ongoing. A total of more than 200 publications were reviewed for the 2015 and 2016 White Papers together and no major challenges to the findings and assumptions of the 2013 Report were found. The approach taken was as follows: for each thematic area, the White Paper first recalls what the 2013 Report had concluded on the subject, and then introduced the review of new information against that. This helps convey the relevance and importance of the new material, and also highlights areas for future research. All the aforementioned publications are available for cost-free download from the UNSCEAR website (www.unscear.org), in English and Japanese.

2015 White Paper

For the 2015 White Paper, updated scientific information of interest to the research community was identified. In the area of radionuclide releases into the atmosphere, refinements in release estimates had been published; they were broadly consistent with the UNSCEAR 2013 Report, but provided more detail on the pattern of atmospheric release with time and used new information on radiation dose rates and levels of radionuclides in the environment. The Committee reconfirmed that radionuclides other than radiocesium and radioiodine did not contribute significantly to human exposure. Except possibly for evacuees, the new publications had no impact on the estimates of doses published in the 2013 Report.

Regarding radionuclide releases into water, some publications provided an improved understanding of the mechanisms of dispersion in coastal waters, but the main findings of the UNSCEAR 2013 Report remained valid.

With respect to exposures of the general public, the doses decreased substantially after 2011, as foreseen. The doses from food were confirmed to be small, and from the inhalation of resuspended radiocesium negligible. Whole-body measurements had been published that supported an emerging consensus that doses from food consumption may have been much lower than estimated in 2013 using food and deposition measurements combined with modeling. Nevertheless, because external exposure dominates, it was concluded that the total doses are not affected significantly. Several papers of scientific interest have been published on migration of radiocesium in various environments and on its transfer to specific foodstuffs in Japan; although they do not affect the total exposure estimates, these issues are worthy of future scientific study.

Reflecting on the future outlook for exposures, it is known that dose rates vary with location, age, and behavior of the individuals exposed, that the exposure to radioiodine finished within the first few months, that the main focus now is on long-lived radiocesium, and that exposures in the first year were the highest with ongoing low exposures in later years. These findings are completely consistent with the UNSCEAR 2013 Report.

The group also reviewed new publications related to exposure of workers. While some significant changes to the estimates of doses to some workers had been published, the main findings of the UNSCEAR 2013 Report were unaffected. It was concluded that a fuller analysis of the data and methodologies used to reevaluate doses in Japan was needed.

Regarding the health implications of the radiation exposure of workers and the public, the group concluded that the 2013 Report's findings remained valid. New published information gave added weight to conclusions on the screening effect for thyroid cancer in children. The group decided to keep abreast of ongoing research in this area, and the Committee encouraged greater access to health data for emergency workers and screened people.

In particular, the group considered information on the incidence of thyroid cancer among children. The 2013 Report had concluded that, theoretically, there was a small increased risk of thyroid cancer among children most exposed to radioiodine in the first several weeks after the accident. As part of the 2015 White Paper, electronic attachments provide calculations analyzing the statistical power of a hypothetical epidemiological study designed to detect an increased incidence in thyroid cancer among this group. These calculations indicated that an increased incidence of thyroid cancer would theoretically be discernible (to a rate 30% higher than the normal rate) assuming (1) the health of 3-year-old girls was followed completely for 50 years, (2) the average thyroid doses were greater than those to a control group by some 20 mGy, and (3) the probability of thyroid cancer induction after the Fukushima accident was assumed pessimistically to be 2.5 times the current best estimate of the probability derived from previous studies. However, detecting and confirming an increase in the reported incidence of thyroid cancer would be severely complicated by the well-known phenomenon of increased detection that occurs with any screening program. The Fukushima Health Management Survey uses highly sensitive ultrasound techniques to screen for nodules, cysts, and cancers of the thyroid. Small thyroid cancers were detected early on in the screened population that would not normally have been detected, despite the reported excess cancers occurring too soon to be due to radiation from the accident. The intensive and highly sensitive screening has detected these small existing cancers, and thus the incidence rates appear to rise, even though they are not due to radiation exposure. This is supported by the observation that the age distribution of the thyroid cancers does not match that seen after the Chernobyl accident—one of the most comprehensive and well-documented accidents in terms of radiological impact.

With respect to the doses and effects for nonhuman biota, the findings of the 2013 Report were broadly supported. The Committee encouraged more field studies, as most available information was based on laboratory work. It suggested that such field studies be designed to analyze the impact of exposure to ionizing radiation and be multidisciplinary in nature.

In the 2015 White Paper, the Committee identified areas in which scientific research would be warranted: in-depth studies of wet deposition and improved source term modeling; models of external exposure for various building types and different seasons, and follow-up of the impact of remediation; detailed evaluation of doses to evacuees based on the latest source term estimates; studies of the migration of cesium in urban, agricultural, and forest environments and the transfer to cultivated and wild foodstuffs, and parameters related to food distribution and consumption habits for those foodstuffs; assessment of doses to lens of the eye for workers; quantification of the impact of screening (collecting thyroid screening data from nonexposed young people, if this were ethically appropriate); analysis of thyroid cancer data by age and sex; and the resolution of anomalies in data reported on effects on plants and animals.

2016 White Paper

The 2016 White Paper reviewed scientific publications available up to the end of 2015. A significant publication for this period was that of the International Atomic Energy Agency, a report which describes the accident and its causes, evolution, and consequences based on data and information from a large number of sources. That report and most of the new publications again confirmed the main assumptions and findings of the UNSCEAR 2013 Report. The scope of the reviews was also extended to specifically include the transfer of radionuclides in terrestrial and freshwater environments. For the second year onwards, the Committee had modeled transfers through these environments to estimate doses to the public from foodstuffs. In the 2016 White Paper, the Committee focused on the transfer pathways for radiocesium (which is the dominant radionuclide). New information was reviewed on radiocesium fixation and migration in soil; radiocesium transfer from soil to crops and, finally, transfer to food products that had not been considered in the 2013 Report. While there is new information that has become available on transfers of radioactive material in soils and into foods specific to Japanese conditions, the overall effect on predicted doses from food consumption from the second year onwards has been minor and the 2016 White Paper thus concluded that the main findings of the 2013 Report remained valid.

Several publications identified areas for which further analysis or more conclusive evidence from research was needed.

RELEVANCE OF OUTREACH ACTIVITIES

While the solid scientific and technical assessment of the accident has been the fundamental objective of the Committee, these publications are of little value if they are not brought to the attention of people who can use them. Thus, in parallel with the technical work, the secretariat has implemented an outreach strategy for the UNSCEAR 2013 report and subsequent White Papers.

Following the triple tragedy, media reports and other anecdotal evidence suggested that the Japanese public would welcome independent scientific information on the radiological impact of the accident. With the support of Fukushima Prefecture, the secretariat organized the first outreach/focus group events in Fukushima City and Koriyama City in September 2014, and has since organized other such events in Iwaki and Minamisoma (in February 2016) and most recently in Aizuwakamatsu (in November 2016).

The strategy has been to target these events at so-called "multipliers" or "influencers"—these are individuals who engage regularly with people directly affected by the accident, such as teachers and academics, medical staff and professionals, social services staff, animal welfare experts, and municipal officers. The rationale is that they are a repository of the concerns of the local populations and would benefit from being able to aggregate these concerns and discuss them with independent experts in the context of the Committee's publications. In turn, the Committee benefited by learning about the concerns of the most affected populations.

The format of the events has typically been a short presentation by a panel composed of the Committee's lead experts in the relevant subject areas, followed by a robust question and answer session. All proceedings are consecutively translated into Japanese and even the slides are bilingual.

The purpose of these events is twofold: (1) to reinforce the seriousness of the Committee's commitment to assess and communicate levels and effects of radiation exposure after the accident and, (2) to provide unbiased, independent scientific information to the public.

Support and interest in these events has been overwhelmingly positive (see Fig. 19.1), and reaffirms that interest in the issue, even 5 years after the tragedy, is alive. The presence of the experts, who engage with the audience and answer questions with hard facts that people can use, has been much appreciated, as is evident with the length of the question and answer sessions that have sometimes gone on for well over an hour. Questions in past events have ranged from whether driving children to school will provide shielding, to whether local produce was safe to eat.

To further assist communication, these events were supported by fact sheets in Japanese and by voluntary financial contributions to the

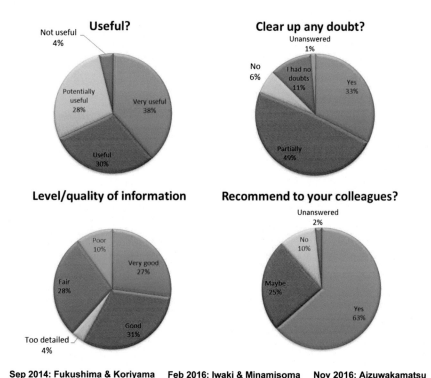

Sep 2014: Fukushima & Koriyama   Feb 2016: Iwaki & Minamisoma   Nov 2016: Aizuwakamatsu

Figure 19.1 Feedback from focus groups 2014–16 (about 500 participants).

UNSCEAR trust fund. Moreover the Committee has a web page dedicated to the Fukushima accident (also in Japanese), as well as a short film of its activities. All are available at http://www.unscear.org/unscear/en/fukushima.html.

Although not directly focused on the accident, the UNSCEAR secretariat has also fostered an update of a basic booklet for the public on "radiation effects and sources" published by UNEP. This provides background information on sources of exposure to radiation and typical levels, as well as an overview of the effects on human health and the environment—a Japanese translation is also in the pipeline.

FUKUSHIMA COMPARED WITH CHERNOBYL

The accident at the Fukushima-Daiichi nuclear power station is regularly compared with that at Chernobyl Unit 4, but the two are very different. The airborne release and ground deposition in Japan of the most radiologically significant radionuclides is perhaps 10% of that at Chernobyl. The Fukushima release includes only volatile nuclides (iodine, tellurium, and cesium) in contrast to the releases from Chernobyl which also included refractory elements (including plutonium). The contaminated areas of Japan are much smaller than the areas contaminated after the Chernobyl accident; however the areas in Japan have much higher population densities. Prompt precautionary protection actions substantially reduced the population doses in Japan. Both individual and collective doses to the Japanese public are much less than 10% of those at Chernobyl; and doses to the thyroid are much smaller still, because of the difference in season and of countermeasures implementation. No acute radiation effects among the general public or workers were observed after the Fukushima accident, in contrast to deaths and injuries among the emergency workers at Chernobyl; and it is unlikely that increasing cancer rates that could be attributed to radiation exposure will be detected after Fukushima, in contrast to the increased incidence of thyroid cancer among those exposed by the Chernobyl accident as children.

The Committee has followed the Chernobyl accident over the past 30 years and has published three major reports—in 1988 (UNSCEAR, 1988), 2000 (UNSCEAR, 2000), and 2008 (UNSCEAR, 2008a). Moreover in the last 10 years, it has published many specialized annexes that have information pertinent to assessing the Fukushima accident, including: the 2013 annex on effects of radiation exposure on children (UNSCEAR, 2013b); the 2012 annexes on the ability to attribute effects to radiation exposure and inference of risk, and uncertainty in cancer risk estimates (UNSCEAR, 2012); the 2008 annex on the effects of ionizing radiation on nonhuman biota (UNSCEAR, 2008b); and the 2006 annexes on epidemiological studies of radiation in cancer, and on epidemiological evaluation of cardiovascular disease and other noncancer diseases following radiation exposure (UNSCEAR, 2008a).

Of interest, at this year's session of the Committee, the secretariat was requested to prepare a short paper that updates and evaluates thyroid cancer data in regions affected by the Chernobyl accident, for discussion at the next session at the end of May 2017.

CONCLUSION

In summary, since estimated doses received by the Japanese public were low, the radiation impact is also expected to be low. Cancer rates are likely to remain stable—it is unlikely that any increase in cancer rates due to radiation exposure would be discernible. The Committee has established a simple, robust, and effective mechanism to follow-up on the accident, and is committed to monitor and analyze the issues, and to bring its findings to Japan and the people affected, with a view to helping them better understand the scientific facts surrounding the situation in which they unfortunately find themselves, and alleviate any unnecessary concerns.

REFERENCES

Action plan for occupational radiation protection, prepared by IAEA and ILO, GOV/2003/47-GC(47)/7 Annex 2.

Developments since the 2013 UNSCEAR Report on the levels and effects of radiation exposure due to the nuclear accident following the great east-Japan earthquake and tsunami (United Nations, 2015). <http://www.unscear.org/unscear/en/publications/Fukushima_WP2015.html>.

Developments since the 2013 UNSCEAR Report on the levels and effects of radiation exposure due to the nuclear accident following the great east-Japan earthquake and tsunami (United Nations, 2016). <http://www.unscear.org/unscear/en/publications/Fukushima_WP2016.html>.

Draft plan of activities on the radiation protection of the environment, IAEA, GOV/2005/45.

Para 15 of Report of the United Nations Scientific Committee on the Effects of Atomic Radiation to the sixty-eighth session of the General Assembly, Document A/68/46 available on <http://www.unscear.org/docs/GAreports/A-68-46_e_V1385727.pdf>.

Resolution 913 (X), adopted 3 December 1955, available on UNSCEAR website at <http://www.unscear.org/unscear/en/general_assembly.html#Resolution%20913%20(X)>.

UNSCEAR, 1958. Report (http://www.unscear.org/unscear/en/publications/1958.html) and the UNSCEAR 1962 Report (http://www.unscear.org/unscear/en/publications/1962.html) laid the scientific grounds on which the partial test ban treaty was negotiated and signed in 1963.

UNSCEAR, 2012. Report Annex A: Attributing health effects to ionizing radiation exposure and inferring risks and Annex B: Uncertainties in risk estimates for radiation-induced cancer (United Nations, 2015). <http://www.unscear.org/unscear/en/publications/2012.html>.

UNSCEAR governing principles were approved at the sixty-first session of UNSCEAR (Vienna, 21–25 July 2014), amended at the sixty-second session (Vienna, 1–5 June 2015), available on UNSCEAR website at <http://www.unscear.org/unscear/en/about_us/governingprinciples.html>.

UNSCEAR, 1988. Report Annex D: "Exposures from the Chernobyl accident" (United Nations, 1988). <http://www.unscear.org/docs/publications/1988/UNSCEAR_1988_Annex-D.pdf>.

UNSCEAR, 2000. Report Vol. II Annex J: Exposures and effects of the Chernobyl accident (United Nations, 2000). <http://www.unscear.org/docs/publications/2000/UNSCEAR_2000_Annex-J.pdf> (United Nations, 2000).

UNSCEAR, 2006. Report Vol I, Annex A: Epidemiological studies of radiation and cancer; and Annex B: Epidemiological evaluation of cardiovascular disease and other non-cancer diseases following radiation exposure (United Nations, 2008). <http://www.unscear.org/unscear/en/publications/2006_1.html>.

UNSCEAR, 2008a. Report Vol II, Annex C: Radiation exposures in accidents; Annex D: Health effects due to radiation from the Chernobyl accident); Annex E:Effects of ionizing radiation on non-human biota. (United Nations, 2011). <http://www.unscear.org/docs/publications/2008/UNSCEAR_2008_Report_Vol.II.pdf>.

UNSCEAR, 2008b. Report Vol II, Annex E-Effects of ionizing radiation on non-human biota (United Nations, 2011). <http://www.unscear.org/docs/publications/2008/UNSCEAR_2008_Report_Vol.II.pdf>.

UNSCEAR, 2013a. Report Vol. I, Annex A: "Levels and effects of radiation exposure due to the nuclear accident after the 2011 great east-Japan earthquake and tsunami" (United Nations, 2014). <http://www.unscear.org/unscear/en/publications/2013_1.html>.

UNSCEAR, 2013b. Report Vol. I, Annex B: "Effects of radiation exposure of children". (United Nations, 2013). <http://www.unscear.org/docs/publications/2013/UNSCEAR_2013_Report_Vol.II.pdf>.

FURTHER READING

International action plan for the radiological protection of patients, prepared by IAEA in consultation with WHO, PAHO, and UNSCEAR, GOV/2002/36-GC(46)/12.

UNSCEAR, 2006. Report Vol I, Annex A: Epidemiological studies of radiation and cancer; and Annex B: Epidemiological evaluation of cardiovascular disease and other non-cancer diseases following radiation exposure (United Nations, 2008). <http://www.unscear.org/unscear/en/publications/2006_1.html>.

CHAPTER 20

The Radiological Consequences of the Fukushima Dai'ichi NPP Accident: Estimates From the Group of Experts Convened by the International Atomic Energy Agency

Abel J. González
Argentine Nuclear Regulatory Authority, Buenos Aires, Argentina

INTRODUCTION

A number of international estimates have been reported on the radiological consequences of the accident at the Fukushima Dai'ichi Nuclear Power Plant on March 11, 2011 (hereinafter referred to as "the accident"). They include those issued by the World Health Organization (WHO, 2012, 2013) and by the United Nations Scientific Committee on the Effects of Atomic Radiation, (UNSCEAR, 2015). The International Atomic Energy Agency (IAEA) issued an all-inclusive report on the accident (IAEA, 2015), which describes the accident comprehensively and inter alia presents a wide-ranging evaluation of the consequences building upon those previous estimates.

THE IAEA REPORT

The IAEA report consists of a main document supported by five broad technical volumes. It has been issued in the six official languages of the United Nations and in Japanese and its full corpus in English is composed of 1254 pages and 311 figures; the main document is supported by 246 references. It is the result of an extensive international collaborative effort involving five working groups including about 180 experts from 42 IAEA Member States and several international bodies (The 2012 56th regular session of the IAEA General Conference was informed that the Agency would prepare an authoritative, factual, and balanced assessment, addressing the causes and consequences of the

Thyroid Cancer and Nuclear Accidents. DOI: http://dx.doi.org/10.1016/B978-0-12-812768-1.00020-4

accident, and the lessons learned. On May 14, 2015, a definitive report on the accident was submitted to the consideration of the IAEA Board of Governors and then released at the 2015 59th session of the IAEA General Conference. For the preparation of the report in-kind contributions were received from Argentina, Australia, Belarus, Brazil, Canada, China, Cuba, the Czech Republic, Finland, France, Germany, Ghana, Iceland, India, Indonesia, Israel, Italy, Japan, the Republic of Korea, Malaysia, Mexico, Morocco, the Netherlands, New Zealand, Norway, Pakistan, Philippines, Poland, the Russian Federation, Slovakia, South Africa, Spain, Sweden, Switzerland, the Syrian Arab Republic, Turkey, Ukraine, the United Arab Emirates, the United Kingdom, the United Republic of Tanzania, the United States of America, the European Commission, the Food and Agriculture Organization of the United Nations, the International Commission on Radiological Protection (ICRP), the International Labour Organization, the International Nuclear Safety Group, the OECD Nuclear Energy Agency, UNSCEAR, the World Association of Nuclear Operators, and the World Meteorological Organization.).

Based on the evaluation of data and information available at the time, the report provides a description of the accident and its causes, evolution, and consequences, and also highlights the main observations and lessons.

The report describes the accident, including the initiating event and response and the accident progression and stabilization efforts, and addresses nuclear safety considerations, including the vulnerability of the plant to external events, the application of the defense in depth concept and the failures to fulfill fundamental safety functions.

The report also considers emergency preparedness and response issues such as the initial response to the accident and the related protection measures for emergency workers and the public, the transition from the emergency phase to the recovery phase, and the response including the international framework for emergency preparedness and response.

The report describes off-site remediation measures of areas affected by the accident, including the establishment of a legal and regulatory framework for remediation, the remediation strategy adopted, and the actual progress in remediation. The on-site stabilization and preparations for decommissioning are also portrayed in the report, including the relevant strategic plans, the preparations for decommissioning, the management of contaminated water, the removal of spent fuel and fuel debris, and the decommissioning end state for the site. Special attention is given to the management of contaminated material and radioactive waste and to the community revitalization and stakeholder engagement, including a panorama of the significant socioeconomic consequences of the accident.

The report finally addresses the international response to the accident, including two Ministerial Conferences on Nuclear Safety (which were held in Vienna and Fukushima), the subsequent IAEA Action Plan on Nuclear Safety, relevant meetings of the Contracting Parties to the Convention on Nuclear Safety, including the Extraordinary Meeting and the Sixth Review Meeting of the Contracting Parties, and (fundamentally!) the relevant 2015 Diplomatic Conference that adopted the *Vienna Declaration on Nuclear Safety*.

However, for the purposes of the Fifth International Expert Symposium in Fukushima, the relevant part of the IAEA report is the estimates of the radiological consequences of the accident by the group of experts convened by the IAEA for that purpose; these are briefly described hereinafter.

ESTIMATES OF THE RADIOLOGICAL CONSEQUENCES
Radioactivity in the Environment
The accident released huge amounts of radionuclides to the environment, the characteristics of which have been assessed by many organizations using different models. In the early phase of the accident, the noble gases krypton-85 (^{85}Kr) and xenon-133 (^{133}Xe), with half-lives of 10.76 years and 5.25 days, respectively, contributed to external exposure from the plume of the atmospheric releases. The short-lived iodine-131 (^{131}I), with a half-life of 8.02 days, contributed to the equivalent doses to the thyroid gland if ingested or inhaled. The longer-lived cesium-134 (^{134}Cs) and cesium-137 (^{137}Cs), with half-lives of 2.06 years and 30.17 years, respectively, contributed to both equivalent doses and effective doses through external and internal exposure. Radionuclides of strontium, ruthenium, and some actinides (e.g., plutonium) were also released in varying amounts. While ^{131}I decays relatively quickly, it can give rise to relatively high equivalent doses to the thyroid gland.

In some areas, ^{137}Cs may continue to be present in the environment, and without remediation it could remain a contributor to effective doses to individuals.

Estimates of the most significant releases are as follows.

For the atmospheric releases:

- 6000–12,000 PBq of ^{133}Xe, or 500–15,000 PBq, if early estimates are included in the evaluation (noble gases were a significant part of the early releases);
- 100–400 PBq of ^{131}I or 90–700 PBq if early estimates are included; and,
- 7–20 PBq of ^{137}Cs, or 7–50 PBq, if early estimates are included.

For the direct releases and discharges into the sea:

- 10–20 PBq of ^{131}I; and,
- 1–6 PBq of ^{137}Cs (but some assessments reported estimates of 2.3–26.9 PBq)

(These releases are estimated to be approximately one-tenth of the releases from the accident of the Chernobyl NPP in 1986.)

Most of the atmospheric releases were blown eastward by the prevailing winds, therefore mainly depositing onto and dispersing within the North Pacific Ocean. Uncertainties in estimations of the amount and composition of the radioactive substances released were difficult to resolve for reasons that included the lack of monitored data on the deposition of the atmospheric releases on the ocean. Moreover, the precise movement of radionuclides in the ocean was difficult to assess by measurements alone and a number of oceanic transport models had to be used to estimate the oceanic dispersion.

While the easterly direction toward the ocean dominated the releases, the atmospheric discharges that took place on 12, 14, and 15 March were blown over land and significant radionuclides, notably ^{131}I, ^{134}Cs, and ^{137}Cs were deposited on the ground. The total deposition of long-lived ^{137}Cs on the land surface of Japan was estimated to have been around 2–3 PBq. The largest deposits were found to the northwest of the Fukushima Daiichi NPP. Presented by order of magnitude, the deposition levels at the most affected areas were of the order of 10,000,000 Bq/m^2 and many areas had levels of around

1,000,000 Bq/m^2. The distribution of deposits for the whole affected area of Fukushima Prefecture was found to be inhomogeneous, and the levels immediately outside the most affected areas in Fukushima Prefecture were around 10,000 Bq/m^2. While some other regions of Japan show elevated deposition levels, the levels attributable to the accident in most of Japan were generally lower than around 1000 Bq/m^2.

The highest levels of deposited ^{131}I exceeded 3,000,000 Bq/m^2 immediately after the accident but, owing to the short physical half-life of ^{131}I, the levels decreased rapidly and are now no longer measurable.

In the affected areas, radionuclides released were found in some consumer products and other items in daily use by individuals and households, such as food, drinking water, and some nonedible products. However, restrictions were established after the accident, on 21 March, by the Japanese authorities to prevent the consumption of drinking water and food containing radionuclides at levels that were higher than provisional regulation values. After April 2012, all drinking water in Japan was found to be below WHO guidance values. With rare exceptions, the levels of radionuclides in food available on the market did not exceed those established in the *Codex Alimentarius*, which are applicable to international trade.

Protection of People Against Radiation Exposure

People were exposed to radiation attributable to the releases from the accident through a number of different exposure pathways. Radiation doses incurred by people were estimated, initially by modeling and/or environmental and later by personal measurements, through the various exposure pathways. These estimates and measurements were then used for the protection of people, the main actions being measures of sheltering, evacuation, and relocation of the affected people.

The international protection standards applicable at the time of the accident had been issued in 1996 and were based on recommendations from the ICRP issued in 1990. At the time of the accident, these standards were being revised to reflect new ICRP recommendations issued in 2007, which provided a framework for dose reference levels for protection purposes. For the highest planned residual dose from a radiological emergency, they recommended reference levels that could be greater than 20 mSv of either acute or annual dose, but not more than

100 mSv. The Japanese regulatory body chose to apply the lower reference level of 20 mSv/year for public protection.

Some protective actions were very difficult for the authorities and extremely demanding for the affected individuals and communities. Sheltering and evacuation were particularly disruptive for around 160,000 people who were isolated from their communities and had access to only limited supplies to meet their daily needs. The initial evacuation led to crowded conditions in shelters. People were eventually relocated, but their normal living conditions were greatly affected. Employment and participation in community activities were limited. Their prospects were uncertain and planning for the future was very difficult.

As far as occupational protection is concerned, the Japanese regulations were consistent with international recommendations and standards, which establish a dose limit for occupational exposure as an effective dose of 20 mSv/year, averaged over 5 years, and 50 mSv in any single year. For emergency workers, a limiting effective dose criterion of 100 mSv was in place. This criterion had to be temporarily increased by the Japanese authorities to a dose limit of 250 mSv for the emergency workers who were within 30 km of the Fukushima Daiichi NPP until December 16, 2011. Some shortcomings occurred in the implementation of occupational radiation protection requirements, including during the early monitoring and recording of radiation doses of emergency workers, in the availability and use of some protective equipment and in associated training.

The Radiation Exposure Incurred by People

The radiation doses caused by exposure attributable to the accident, which were estimated by the experts, built upon those previous estimates by WHO and UNSCEAR but they also benefited from the availability of additional information, particularly from the Fukushima Health Management Survey and data on direct measurements of dose to people and radiation in the environment. The dose estimates for members of the public by WHO and UNSCEAR were constrained by limited availability of direct radiation measurements of individual doses incurred by people and were mainly made using dose assessment models based on environmental conditions. The WHO estimates were generally higher than those of UNSCEAR primarily because they were early theoretical dose projections based on very limited data following the accident. The early assessments of radiation doses used environmental monitoring and dose estimation models, resulting in some overestimations. The experts' estimates included personal monitoring data delivered by the local authorities, which provided more robust information on the actual individual doses incurred and their distribution.

This is a relevant characteristic of the experts' dose estimates, namely that they were based not only on theoretical models but also on real measurements on people. Moreover, the collected data were subject to a comprehensive statistical analysis. The values of recorded variable doses were classified according to their frequency distribution, by binning the whole range of data into histograms, which were then normalized. When sufficient data were available, with the bin intervals becoming very small, the histogram tends towards a smooth probability density function describing the relative likelihood for the dose incurred by people having a given value. Thus, the log-normal distribution of doses was estimated, namely the probability distribution of dose, whose logarithm is normally distributed, where the log-normal probability density function is symmetrical with respect to the maximum only when displayed as a function of the logarithm of the dose. The log-normal probability density function was then integrated, resulting in a log-normal cumulative probability function, describing the likelihood that a dose with a given probability distribution will be found to have a value less than or equal to the value. The log-normal cumulative probability functions were plotted in coordinate planes of abscissas representing the dose calibrated logarithmically versus ordinates representing the cumulative probability calibrated as a normal function and it was compared with an expected straight line to ensure the robustness of the data.

In the short term, the most significant contributors to the exposure of the public were external exposure from radionuclides in the plume and deposited on the ground and internal exposure of the thyroid gland, due to the intake of ^{131}I, and internal exposure of other organs and tissues, mainly due to the intake of ^{134}Cs and ^{137}Cs. In the long term, the most important contributor to the exposure of the public will be external radiation from the deposited ^{137}Cs.

A statistical analysis was undertaken of individual effective doses due to external radiation in various municipalities of Fukushima

Prefecture that had been estimated by using data collected by the Fukushima Health Management Survey. External doses in the first 4 months were, on average, lower among the populations in the 20-km zone than those from locations outside this area, as a consequence of the early evacuation of this zone, which in addition showed wider distributions than those for locations outside the zone due to the evacuation of members of the same community to different locations and often further movements leading to differences in the doses received. In sum, from the analysis, the result of mean doses, and dose range for a confidence limit of 95%, for various cities of the Fukushima Prefecture, was as follows: Futaba, mean, 0.24 mSv, range, 0.022–2.7 mSv; Kawauchi, mean, 0.4 mSv, range, 0.07–2.3 mSv; Naraha, mean, 0.11 mSv, range, 0.01–1.1 mSv; Okuma, mean 0.28 mSv, range, 0.027–2.9 mSv; Minamisoma, mean, 0.48 mSv, range, 0.11–2.2 mSv; Tomioka, mean, 0.26 mSv, range, 0.036–2 mSv; Namie, mean 0.37 mSv, range, 0.035–3.9 mSv; Date, mean, 1.1 mSv, range, 0.41–2.9 mSv; Katsurao, mean, 0.62 mSv, range, 0.16–2.5 mSv; Fukushima, mean 1.3 mSv, range 0.6–2.6 mSv; Kawamata, mean, 1.1 mSv, range 0.32–3.6 mSv; Iitate, mean, 3.1 mSv, range 0.96–10 mSv; Nihonmatsu, mean, 1.5 mSv, range 0.87–2.6 mSv; Iwaki, mean, 0.097 mSv, range 0.015–0.62 mSv; and Tamura, mean, 0.46 mSv, range, 0.15–1.4 mSv.

But the more important corroboration of individual doses from external radiation was provided by the data on individual monitoring using personal dosimeters. When personal monitoring data became available, they allowed comparison between the two different approaches, using assumptions about people's habits and models, to estimate the effective dose incurred versus monitoring the actual personal dose equivalent incurred, confirming that modeled doses are usually overestimations compared with actually incurred doses (this had been also observed during the dose assessments in the aftermath of the Chernobyl accident). These estimates indicate that the effective doses incurred by members of the public were low and generally comparable with the range of effective doses incurred due to global levels of natural background radiation. Probability distribution of monitored personal dose equivalents of members of the public during 2011 provided by the Government of Japan for two municipalities in the affected area for which annualized data were available showed personal dose equivalents averaging below 1 mSv/year, providing 95% confidence that individuals who incurred effective doses in those municipalities sustained doses below 5 mSv.

These estimates indicate that the external effective doses incurred by members of the public were low and generally comparable with the range of effective doses incurred due to global levels of natural background radiation.

Regarding the internal exposure by adults, the monitored levels of radioactivity intake were generally lower than the very low detection limits of the whole-body counters, indicating little or no intake of radionuclides into the body. Where it was possible to convert measured intakes to effective dose, making assumptions about the timing and nature of the intake, the vast majority of estimates of the committed effective dose were less than 1 mSv and the estimated effective dose commitment was reported to be lower than around 1 mSv in 99% of the residents. However, many whole-body counting measurements were carried out several months after the accident and are therefore often only applicable to ^{134}Cs and ^{137}Cs and not to the short-lived ^{131}I, therefore making definitive judgments on internal exposure difficult. However, in few measurements of ^{131}I the highest estimated thyroid absorbed dose was 20 mGy (i.e., a thyroid equivalent dose of 20 mSv), with a corresponding effective dose of around 1 mSv.

The intake by children of ^{131}I and the subsequent doses to their thyroid glands and their uncertainties were a particular concern. However, the typical intake of ^{131}I via cow's milk was very low following the accident, owing to a number of factors, as follows: (1) dairy practices in Japan, such as generally sheltering cattle, prevented the ingestion of ^{131}I by dairy cows; (2) the intake of ^{131}I via milk was also limited by the relatively low contribution of milk to the diet of infants and by the strict restrictions on the consumption of milk imposed by the authorities following the accident; and, (3) while there were alternative ^{131}I ingestion pathways, such as the consumption of leafy vegetables and drinking water, especially in the very early period following the release, the prompt restrictions on drinking water and food limited the intake via these pathways.

Fortunately, therefore, as a result of these factors, the reported thyroid equivalent doses of children appear to have been low. Thyroid equivalent doses to some children were estimated by monitoring levels of external radiation from ^{131}I activity in the gland, which were measured on the skin, near the thyroid, of children from areas where thyroid doses were predicted to be high. A limited number of these direct measurements were reported for the weeks following the accident. The results of one study, in which 1080 measurements were made on children aged 1−15 years showed that the highest ambient dose equivalent rate measured near the thyroid of 1-year-old children was 0.0001 mSv/h, which would be consistent with an absorbed dose to the thyroid of approximately 50 mGy (a thyroid equivalent dose of 50 mSv). It was reported that thyroid equivalent doses, in the evacuation zone, were lower than around 10 mSv in 95.7% of children (with a maximum of 43 mSv). In sum, the experts concluded that it is likely that all doses were lower than the generic optimized intervention value for iodine prophylaxis of 100 mGy of avertable committed absorbed dose to the thyroid due to radioiodine established in the 1996 international standards and also lower than the projected dose of 50 mSv in the first 7 days for iodine thyroid blocking established in the revised international standards as generic criteria for protective actions and other response actions in an emergency. In comparison, the absorbed doses by thyroid of children following the Chernobyl accident ranged up to several thousand mGy, namely nearly 100−1000 times higher.

As far as occupational doses are concerned, the effective doses incurred by most of the around 23,000 emergency workers who had been involved in emergency operations by December 2011 were below the occupational dose limits in Japan. A total of 174 emergency workers exceeded the original criterion for emergencies and six emergency workers exceeded the temporarily revised effective dose criterion in an emergency established by the Japanese authority. No workers exceeded the relevant international effective dose for emergencies in subsequent years, and only one worker exceeded the occupational annual effective dose limit for normal operations.

The Health Effects Attributable to the Accidental Exposure

The experts underlined that no early radiation-induced health effects were observed among workers or members of the public that could be attributed to the accident. While the latency time for late radiation health effects can be decades (and therefore it is not possible to discount the potential occurrence of such effects among an exposed population by observations a few years after exposure), however, the experts estimated (in agreement with UNSCEAR) that, given the low levels of doses reported among members of the public, no discernible increased incidence of radiation-related health effects were expected among exposed members of the public and their descendants. The experts however warned that, among the group of few workers who received high effective doses, an increased risk of cancer could be expected in the future although it would be indiscernible.

The experts highlighted that, because the reported thyroid doses incurred by children were generally low, an increase in pediatric thyroid cancer attributable to the accident was unlikely.

The expert noted that prenatal radiation effects have not been observed and are not expected to occur, given that the reported doses are well below the threshold at which these effects may take place. They also noted that unwanted terminations of pregnancy attributable to the radiological situation have not been reported. Concerning the possibility of parents' exposures resulting in hereditary effects in their descendants, the experts concluded (in agreement with UNSCEAR) that although demonstrated in animal studies, an increase in the incidence of hereditary effects in human populations cannot at present be attributed to radiation exposure.

The experts emphasized that psychological conditions were reported among the population affected by the nuclear accident. However, since a number of these people had suffered the combined impacts of a major earthquake and a devastating tsunami as well as the accident, it was concluded that it was difficult to assess to what extent these effects could be attributed to the nuclear accident alone. Notwithstanding, associated psychological problems were recorded in some vulnerable groups of the affected population, such as increases in anxiety and posttraumatic stress disorders. In agreement with UNSCEAR, the experts estimated that the most important health effect from the accident was on mental and social wellbeing, related to the enormous impact of the earthquake, tsunami, and nuclear accident, and the fear and stigma related to the perceived risk of exposure to ionizing radiation.

The Radiological Consequences for Nonhuman Biota
The experts noted that no observations of direct radiation-induced effects in plants and animals have been reported, although limited

observational studies were conducted in the period immediately after the accident. While there are limitations in the available methodologies for assessing radiological consequences, however, based on previous experience and the levels of radionuclides present in the environment, the experts considered it unlikely that there would be any major radiological consequences for biota populations or ecosystems as a consequence of the accident.

CONCLUSION

The main conclusions on the radiological consequences from the accident from the group of experts convened by the IAEA can be summarized as follows:

1. The radiation doses attributable to the accident that were incurred by members of the public have been fortunately low and the occupational doses were mainly within regulatory limits; therefore,
2. No early radiation-induced health effects were observed among workers or members of the public that could be attributed to the accident, and no discernible increased incidence of radiation-related health effects are expected among exposed members of the public and their descendants; and, in particular,
3. The most important health effect of the accident has been on mental and social wellbeing, related to the enormous impact of the earthquake, tsunami, and the accident, and the fear and stigma related to the perceived risk of exposure to ionizing radiation.

These conclusions are based on the detailed information provided in the report, notably on the real incurred doses, which was not available at the time of the WHO and UNSCEAR reports, and on the estimated psychological consequences, which were neither addressed by WHO nor by UNSCEAR. It is noteworthy that such conclusions are coherent and consistent with the findings previously reported by UNSCEAR to the UN General Assembly.

REFERENCES

IAEA, 2015. International Atomic Energy Agency. The Fukushima Daiichi Accident (Non-serial Publication). Report by the Director General and five technical volume. Subject Classification: 0610-Accident response STI/PUB/1710; (ISBN:978-92-0-107015-9); 1254 pp. 311 figures; IAEA, Vienna, 2015.

UNSCEAR, 2015. United Nations Scientific Committee on the Effects of Atomic Radiation. Sources, Effects and Risks of Ionizing Radiation. Volume 1: Report to the General Assembly and Scientific Annex A: Levels and effects of radiation exposure due to the nuclear accident after the 2011 great east-Japan earthquake and tsunami. UNSCEAR 2013 Report. United Nations sales publication. E.14.IX.1. United Nations, New York, 2014.

WHO, 2012. Preliminary Dose Estimation From the Nuclear Accident After the 2011 Great East Japan Earthquake and Tsunami. World Health Organization (WHO), Geneva.

WHO, 2013. Health Risk Assessment From the Nuclear Accident After the 2011 Great East Japan Earthquake and Tsunami, Based on a Preliminary Dose Estimation. World Health Organization (WHO), Geneva.

Printed in the United States
By Bookmasters